Mexican Americans and Health

¡Sana! ¡Sana!

Second Edition

Adela de la Torre and Antonio Estrada

THE UNIVERSITY OF
ARIZONA PRESS

TUCSON

The University of Arizona Press
www.uapress.arizona.edu

Printed in the United States of America
20   19   18   17   16   15   6   5   4   3   2   1

ISBN-13: 978-0-8165-3157-8 (paper)

Cover designed by Miriam Warren
Cover photo © bowdenimages/istockphoto

Library of Congress Cataloging-in-Publication Data
Torre, Adela de la, author.
   Mexican Americans and health : ¡sana! ¡sana! / Adela de la Torre and Antonio Estrada. —
Second edition.
        pages cm — (The Mexican American experience)
   Includes bibliographical references and index.
   ISBN 978-0-8165-3157-8 (pbk. : alk. paper)
  1. Mexican Americans—Health and hygiene.   2. Mexican Americans—Medical
care.   3. Minorities—Health and hygiene.   4. Minorities—Medical care.   I. Estrada,
Antonio, author.   II. Torre, Adela de la. Mexican Americans and health. Revision of
(manifestation)   III. Title.   IV. Series: Mexican American experience.
   RA448.5.M4T67   2015
   362.10896872073—dc23
                              2014037295

∞ This paper meets the requirements of ANSI/NISO Z39.48-1992 (Permanence of Paper).

Mexican Americans and Health

Second Edition

THE MEXICAN AMERICAN EXPERIENCE

Adela de la Torre, Editor

The Mexican American Experience is a cluster of modular texts designed to provide greater flexibility in undergraduate education. Each book deals with a single topic concerning the Mexican American population. Instructors can create a semester-long course from any combination of volumes or may choose to use one or two volumes to complement other texts. For more information, please visit www.uapress.arizona.edu/textbooks/latino.htm.

Other books in the series:

Mexican Americans and Health
Adela de la Torre and Antonio Estrada

Chicano Popular Culture
Charles M. Tatum

Mexican Americans and the U.S. Economy
Arturo González

Mexican Americans and the Law
Reynaldo Anaya Valencia, Sonia R. García, Henry Flores, and José Roberto Juárez Jr.

Chicana/o Identity in a Changing U.S. Society
Aída Hurtado and Patricia Gurin

Mexican Americans and the Environment
Devon G. Peña

Mexican Americans and the Politics of Diversity
Lisa Magaña

Mexican Americans and Language
Glenn A. Martínez

Chicano and Chicana Literature
Charles M. Tatum

Chicana and Chicano Art
Carlos Francisco Jackson

Immigration Law and the U.S.-Mexico Border
Kevin R. Johnson and Bernard Trujillo

Chicana and Chicano Mental Health
Yvette G. Flores

Mexican Americans and Education
Estela Godinez Ballón

To my family, my daughters, Adelita and Gabriela, my mother, Herminia Domitila, my Tía Tanna, my husband, Stephen, and the memory of my beloved Abuelita Adela. Their constant support and encouragement make all things possible.

—Adela de la Torre

To my wife, Barbara, my children, Charlene, Gloria, and Eric, my father, Antonio, and all my family, who have provided me with endless support and encouragement over the years.

—Antonio Estrada

Sana, sana,
Colita de rana.
Si no sanas hoy,
Sanarás mañana.

Get well, get well,
Little frog tail.
If today you don't get well,
Tomorrow you will be well.

Traditional saying recited to comfort a child while rubbing the site of a pain or injury

CONTENTS

ILLUSTRATIONS

Figures

Tables

ACKNOWLEDGMENTS

This book would not have been possible without the help of several people. We would like to take this opportunity to acknowledge their efforts and thank them for their assistance and participation in this project. First, we would like to thank the undergraduate students at the University of Arizona who conducted the community interviews that are an integral part of this book. They include Carlos R. Acuña, Maria Acuña, Susan Ammouri, Maria G. Broadway, Malala Elston, Brooke E. Felker, Marco A. Gámez, Rori Kelly, Daniel B. Lobato, Norma G. Navarro, Cynthia Nevarez, Olivia Nuñez, Olivia Palacios, Belinda Rodriguez, and Joseph Urbina Jr.

We would also like to extend our thanks to graduate student Rosa Gomez Camacho, who provided leadership and guidance in this second edition of the text. Vikrant Aulakh and Erica Orcutt, both undergraduate students from UC Davis, and Gabriela de la Torre provided significant editorial and research support for this second edition. We would also like to acknowledge Penelope Cray for her excellent editorial assistance for our second edition of this text. Thomas Gelsinon and Kirsteen E. Anderson gave us the benefit of their editorial expertise early on. We would also like to thank cartographers Gary Christopherson and Carol Placchi for developing the original maps for the text (figures 9 through 12). Finally, we would like to acknowledge Kristen A. Buckles for her vision and support for this project.

ACRONYMS USED IN THE TEXT

AAMC	American Association of Medical Colleges
ACA	Affordable Care Act
AFDC	Aid to Families with Dependent Children
AHCCCS	Arizona Health Care Cost Containment System, the Arizona equivalent of Medicaid
AIDS	acquired immunodeficiency syndrome
CDC	Centers for Disease Control and Prevention
DAWN	Drug Abuse Warning Network
DTP	diphtheria-tetanus-pertussis vaccine
EBPI	employer-based private insurance
HHANES	Hispanic Health and Nutrition Examination Survey
HIV	human immunodeficiency virus
HPV	human papillomavirus
HRSA	U.S. Health Resources and Services Administration
IDU	injection drug user
INS	Immigration and Naturalization Service
IPV	intimate partner violence
IRCA	Immigration Reform and Control Act
LEP	limited English proficiency
MSM	men who have sex with men
NCHS	National Center for Health Statistics
NHANES	National Health and Nutrition Examination Survey
NIDA	National Institute on Drug Abuse
NIDDM	non-insulin-dependent diabetes mellitus
NIH	National Institutes of Health
PPACA	Patient Protection and Affordable Care Act
PCP	phenylcyclohexyl piperidine, or angel dust
SAMHSA	Substance Abuse and Mental Health Services Administration
SSA	Social Security Administration

SSI	Supplemental Security Income
STD	sexually transmitted disease
USDA-NIFA	United States Department of Agriculture's National Institute of Food and Agriculture

Mexican Americans and Health

Second Edition

Overview of Health-Care Issues

"I'm Healthy But ..."

Mexican Americans and Health, the inaugural volume in the Mexican American Experience series, is now in its second edition, with updated information directly relevant to understanding the health and health policy issues impacting this large segment of the Latino community. Since this book is intended primarily as an undergraduate textbook, we have tried to make it as accessible as possible. At the end of each chapter, readers will find a set of discussion questions that serve as a review of the key content in the chapter. In addition to source notes and a bibliography listing the print and Internet sources we relied on, we provide a list of suggested readings for anyone wishing to study a topic in more depth. Technical and Spanish-language terms are defined in a glossary at the end of the book. Words that appear in the glossary are in boldface on first reference as a signal to turn to the glossary for a more detailed explanation of that term.

The rapid growth of the Mexican American population and the increasing interest in issues of human diversity has created a need for introductory texts that address critical issues in the Mexican American community. We hope this book will provide insight into a long-neglected subject: the cultural, linguistic, and health policy issues that influence how Mexican Americans access—or fail to access—the U.S. health-care system.

Overview of Health-Care Issues for People of Mexican Origin

Many factors influence the health of the Mexican-origin population of the United States. For example, individual health is intricately related to social and population conditions as well as genetic factors. Although this group shares certain **health status** and access issues with other minorities—African Americans, Native Americans, and Asian Americans—some issues affect people of Mexican descent in distinct ways. Although historical and political-geographical factors affect the overall health status of **Mexican**

Americans, the literature on Mexican American health often ignores these factors. Yet, historical context is how this group defines its identity and its social location within the broader U.S. society. This, in turn, influences how its members enter the health-care system and how they are treated within it.

Elaborating on the issue of identity and social location requires that we understand the deep roots Mexican Americans have in the U.S. Southwest, which for centuries was Mexican territory. These roots predate the incorporation of this region into the United States. Moreover, discrimination, which has influenced the **educational attainment** and **occupational location** of Mexican Americans, is linked to their historical and political incorporation, or lack thereof, within the U.S. Southwest.

With this in mind, the term "Mexican-origin population" includes people who are Mexican **immigrants** as well as **native-born** Mexican Americans. Although other terms such as **Chicano/Chicana** and **Latino/Latina** are often used, they are less specific to the Mexican-origin population based on self-reported U.S. census data. The term "**Hispanic**" is a broader category including other subgroups such as Puerto Ricans, Cubans, Central Americans, and other census-designated Hispanic subgroups. Where possible, we attempt to use data specific to people of Mexican origin. However, these data are available only for certain health-status categories, so we have had to use data from the overall Latino population for some health indicators.

Throughout this text, we also integrate voices of Mexican-origin people to illustrate how their experiences frame health issues. For example, in chapter 1 we will show how decisions about family location contribute to the concentration of Mexican Americans in the Southwest. This is clearly explained by our interviewees Carmen and Marco:

> Actually . . . I didn't have a choice directly as the decision had been made generations before me as to where the family would set root and they did so because the Santa Cruz Valley at that time was very fertile and very green. The river was flowing and the climate was pleasant; it was just an ideal location. (Carmen G., 49)

> I finally met up with my mother and with my brother . . . two or three years after he [my brother] went to San Diego. [I came to the Southwest] because my family was here. I don't know why they chose the Southwest, probably because of proximity [to Mexico]. (Marco G., 28)

The voices of everyday people such as Carmen and Marco will help demonstrate how the Mexican-origin population experiences health and health care, and how their experience is linked to their cultural roots. It is just as important to listen to these voices in the twenty-first century as it was in the twentieth. The voices of the *abuelos, tíos, padres, hermanos,* and *hijos* (grandparents, aunts and uncles, parents, sisters and brothers, and children) to whom you will be introduced offer guidance in the development of health-care strategies that will result in better health for Mexican Americans and the nation as a whole.

We have developed a model that serves as an underlying framework for understanding the most influential factors that affect the health status of Mexican Americans and the way the health-care system responds to this group. The following flowchart illustrates how different components influence the health status of the U.S. Mexican-origin population.

Starting from the left of the diagram, we see how the historical experiences and political-geographical location of the Mexican-origin population influence sociodemographic (social and population) factors such as occupation and immigrant status. These sociodemographic **variables** influence issues of **health-care access**, environmental and behavioral health, and cultural factors, which in turn influence the health status of this group. Genetic factors also play a role in health status, as they do for everyone, but they are not directly influenced by these other factors. An overarching structural element that affects the health status of this group, and other groups, is the U.S. health-care delivery system. Ultimately, this system provides both opportunities and barriers to the Mexican-origin population.

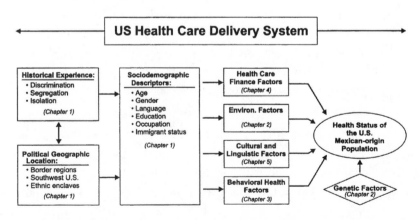

Figure I. Factors influencing the health status of Mexican Americans.

Although constructed independently of the Mexican American community, this system has a profound influence on the group's future social, economic, and health well-being.

The chapter numbers on the diagram indicate where we will discuss each of these important factors. We hope that readers will have, by the end of the book, a broader understanding of the complex issues surrounding the health and health care of the U.S. Mexican-origin population. The following is a brief overview of each chapter.

In chapter 1 we discuss the historical roots and political-geographical concentration of Mexican-origin people in the Southwest and elsewhere. These factors have fostered cultural resiliency and affect the group's perceptions of health care and disease, as well as how they view the dominant society. This chapter also examines socioeconomic status, which is often the main predictor of health status and health-care access. For example, one reason Mexican Americans fare more poorly than the dominant society in terms of jobs and education is that the current demand for cheap labor in the industrial and agricultural sectors of the economy requires the constant flow of immigrant labor, primarily from Mexico. Gracie's childhood memories clearly illustrate this point:

> Being poor, my father never gave it a second thought about taking me to the emergency room. Instead he told my mother to take me to the hospital in the morning. . . . So my mother woke me up. At that time I think I was so exhausted from vomiting and the pain was so strong that I was kicking and I nearly kicked a hole in the wall. . . . Mind you my mother didn't know English so I had to translate for her. So I was coming in and out of consciousness and finally we made it to the hospital, a public hospital in Houston. . . . My mother was holding me in her arms, and if it had not been for the fact that the doctor just happened to be going through the lobby area, and saw me pass out, and noticed the purple lips, I would probably be dead. . . . He realized that my appendix had burst at that moment and quickly rushed me to the emergency room for immediate surgery. (Gracie S., 46)

Much of the recent literature that focuses on health and health-care access examines variables such as educational attainment, poverty status, occupational location, and marital status, as these data explain many of the differences between the health status of the Mexican-origin population and that of other groups. Cultural variables, such as immigrant status and mastery of English, are other strong influences that affect how well individual people of Mexican origin are integrated into the health-care system. Language status, language choice, and linguistic discrimination influence level of education, and ultimately, economic status, which in turn influences health status. Another important factor that differentiates this Latino **subpopulation** is the perceived origin of the discrimination experienced by this group. Unlike other Latino subpopulations, such as Cuban Americans and Central Americans, the experience of racial and ethnic discrimination for the Mexican-origin population is rooted in the historical conquest of the Southwest and the loss of homeland, language, and culture. Making matters worse are the Mexican economic dependency on the U.S. economy and American dependence on low-wage Mexican labor in agriculture and other industries. These factors have created an underclass of immigrants and increased racial tensions and divisions in the Southwest and elsewhere. Thus, it is not surprising to find **racialized** labor markets where the concentration of Mexican immigrants is high. In low-wage sectors, working conditions are often terrible and employee health insurance is not provided, which ultimately has a big effect on the health status of workers. These low-wage sectors include the farm labor market, the non-unionized service sector, and the manufacturing sector. Marco, reflecting on his experiences as a worker in the service sector, states:

> As far as the pay is concerned and the load of work they have to do, it is bullshit.... They are worked to death.... Some of these ladies are going well into their fifties, and they are doing manual labor. I mean it is heavy work. There are times when I leave work, after I've worked a dinner function, and I will walk back to the dishwashing room and it's hot and they have hundreds of dishes and it's two people.... They're understaffed and they are underpaid. (Marco G., 28)

Chapter 2 presents the health status of the Mexican-origin population relative to that of the rest of the population. Despite the low socioeconomic status of many Mexican Americans, there is an interesting phenomenon known as the Mexican American **morbidity** and **mortality** paradox. Even though Mexican-origin individuals have a low socioeconomic status, similar to that of African Americans, morbidity (illness) and mortality (death) data do not reflect the same effects of economic and social disadvantage as for African Americans. This concept has been applied most frequently to childbearing women and mortality rates. Low-income Mexican immigrants have low infant mortality rates and very good birth outcomes, which is not the case for African Americans. Mexican-origin populations also have lower overall mortality rates than do African Americans. Nonetheless, there are health problems that pose concerns for the Mexican-origin community. For children, these include childhood **obesity**, lack of immunizations, and oral health problems. The problem of oral health affects young adults also, as explained by Lily, a twenty-year-old college student:

> I'm healthy, but I know that when it comes to going to the dentist I need to see somebody. And, I know that it's expensive to go. I was in the doctor's office and he said you need to get your wisdom teeth out, but it costs a lot of money and I can't. . . . I even went to talk to someone to see if I could apply for Medicaid . . . just to have backup while at the university. (Lily Q., 20)

The most significant health problems for women are related to prenatal care, preventable cancers such as breast cancer and cervical cancer, and intimate partner violence (IPV). For Mexican-origin workers who have jobs in agriculture, occupational hazards include work-related injuries, pesticide poisoning, heat-related conditions, musculoskeletal disorders, and communicable diseases. Major health problems of the adult population include diabetes, cardiovascular disease (heart disease and heart attack), cancer (in particular colorectal and prostate), substance abuse, and human immunodeficiency disease/acquired immunodeficiency disease (**HIV/AIDS**). In light of these health issues, it is important to develop culturally sensitive, community-based health care for the Mexican-origin population. To do so, we must consider the cultural values of this population. Values such as **machismo, familismo**, and **marianismo** influence care-seeking decisions and treatment of illness.

More recent research on genetic admixture and certain diseases that are prevalent among Mexican Americans suggests an important contribution of Native American genes. Several studies have found a significant association with breast cancer, cardiovascular disease, Type II diabetes, obesity, and asthma. Applied genetic interventions may hold the promise of reducing the incidence of these diseases in future populations of Mexican-origin Latinos.

Chapter 3 discusses the behavioral health issues affecting Mexican Americans. Substance abuse, HIV/AIDS, and violence are major problems, but there are limited data specific to this group. To date, the data indicate that these problems may develop differently in people of Mexican origin than in other Latino/a subpopulations. For example, drug abuse seems to have an early onset in Mexican-origin youth. The peer norms of this group are also somewhat favorable to drug dealing as a source of income, given the limited economic opportunities for Mexican-origin youth as well as their concentration in low-income **ethnic enclaves**.

Acculturation and demographic (population) factors influence the type of drug used and the frequency of use by children and adults. There is conflicting evidence concerning the role of Mexican American cultural identity in drug use. Depending on individual circumstances, it may be risk reducing or risk enhancing. For example, someone who strongly identifies with the Mexican American culture may not use drugs because Mexican values and behavior do not support drug use. However, these values and behaviors conflict with the dominant culture. Thus, the additional stress to conform to the dominant culture while maintaining a strong cultural identity may increase the risk of drug use. This dilemma is exemplified by the identity struggle Marco experienced in his youth:

> When I first arrived, I remember getting beat up and I remember fighting because the kids called me "wetback," "greaser," you name it. I remember going to the principal's office twice a week [because of] a fight. It got to the point where I couldn't attend school anymore. The same situation happened to my brother, but then it stopped. I asked him, "How come no one is beating you up anymore?" He said that one of his teachers had recommended that he tell kids that he was from Spain. Sure enough, I went to school [and said] I was from Spain and I never got busted. It was the coolest thing that anyone had ever heard of . . . so for a long time I was telling kids that I was from Spain and they thought I was pretty cool. But, you know, deep inside I am a Mexican, I am a Chicano, and that was taken away from me. (Marco G., 28)

Other significant factors related to substance abuse include socioeconomic status, peer pressure, and family influence. Confounding these variables is the role of drugs in antisocial or violent behavior. There is a strong correlation between antisocial or violent behavior and drug use. Although a causal relationship is difficult to prove, research suggests that there is also a strong correlation between drug use and juvenile delinquency. Use of certain drugs, such as phenylcyclohexyl piperidine (PCP) and cocaine, is linked to increased aggression and violence. In many Mexican American communities, where there is a high degree of substance abuse, violence within neighborhoods, peer groups, and families is a recurring problem. However, further research is needed to determine the specific relationship between drug use and violence among Mexican American youth.

Important research focusing on injection drug users (IDUs) sheds light on the complex dimensions of substance abuse within the Mexican-origin population. Mexican-origin IDUs have an increased chance of contracting and transmitting HIV and other blood-borne diseases. Their risk is higher because they are more likely than non-IDUs of Mexican-origin to share needles and engage in risky sexual behaviors with partners who may or may not be IDUs.

Substance-abuse issues have resulted in an increase in the number of drug-related emergency room visits among Latinos. In addition, Mexican American youth have less knowledge about sex and HIV prevention than other groups do, yet they are engaging in sex at similar rates. As Ernie, a health educator who works with Latino men, observed: "For a lot of these guys that may have a very *machista* attitude. They will not use condoms . . . that's part of the sexual power."

Understanding cultural nuances such as these is a necessity if we are to develop culturally competent drug abuse intervention programs that address AIDS prevention and education for this community. Again, these approaches must reflect and respect core cultural values such as familismo, **respeto**, and **confianza**.

Chapter 4 presents the problem of health-care access and differential immigrant access to care for the nation's Mexican-origin population. Access is a major factor influencing health-care decisions and treatment of illness. For Mexican Americans, barriers include **financial access** and access to culturally and linguistically competent care. The Mexican-origin population has a disproportionate number and percentage of people who are uninsured. More than one-third have no health insurance, either public or private. This occurs in part because many Mexican Americans have low-wage jobs with few fringe benefits, which prevents them from obtaining health insurance through their employers. Many of these workers are considered **working poor**. That is, until recently, they could not afford private health insurance or qualify for public programs such as **Medicaid**.

Other access issues unique to this population include the roles played by immigration and gender. Mexican immigrants constitute the largest sector of legal and undocumented immigrants in the United States, and they are highly concentrated in ethnic enclaves in the Southwest. Given their low-income status, they often must rely on publicly subsidized programs for their health and overall welfare needs. The backlash from many white non-Latino voters against the growth of the Mexican-origin population in this region has created a hostile environment for this group, despite its enormous productivity in the workplace. This hostility is evidenced by the passage of Arizona's S.B. 1070 in 2010, which provided greater reach for local law enforcement to detain individuals during lawful stops to determine immigration status. Unfortunately, Latinos and other minorities can be singled out for racial profiling as a means for officers to decide which individuals are suspected of being in the United States without proper documentation. People who are stopped by officers would have to show documentation of their legal citizenship or residency, and this would disproportionally apply to Latinos. Although this law was challenged and modified, it nonetheless had a chilling effect on undocumented immigrants' use of services, as fear of apprehension and deportation create barriers to movement to seek needed services. These types of policies, legislative discussions, and initiatives at the state and federal levels often limit *legal* immigrants' use of publicly subsidized services.[1] Similarly, the Patient Protection and Affordable Care Act (PPACA) passed in 2010 and implemented in 2014 prohibits undocumented immigrants from participating in health insurance exchanges (where individuals can acquire health insurance through a government mediated market). Legal immigrants who have not obtained full citizenship status must follow a five-year waiting period before they can participate in these exchanges.

Another important distinction within the Mexican-origin population is women's access to health insurance. Susie eloquently expresses her access problems:

> I have a whole list of things that I need to do. I need to have an eye exam, I need to have a female checkup, I have to have a podiatrist look at my feet. Which they're fine, but it's part of the diabetic thing. . . . If I had insurance I would be able to go to the doctor and I'd be done. . . . My teeth are falling out of my head, literally. I don't go to the dentist because dentists want half of the money up front and I need thousands of dollars of work, but I'm terrified of the dentist. . . . It's a huge issue. (Susie D., 40)

Because many women rely on their spouses for health insurance, marital status is a major predictor of health insurance coverage. This is particularly true for Mexican-origin women because family obligations may interrupt their employment and because they have limited employment opportunities available to them. Since many of these women are employed in the low-tier service sector, which include jobs as domestics and child-care providers, they have limited opportunities to obtain private health-care insurance. Moreover, because they often do not pay into the hospital insurance Part A trust fund (**Medicare**),[2] in their senior years they may find themselves ineligible for Medicare coverage. Lack of financial coverage for postmenopausal women between the ages of fifty and sixty-four is a serious issue. These women are at their greatest risk of not having health insurance during a period when they are most likely to experience chronic diseases such as diabetes, hypertension, and breast cancer. The lack of health care can result in higher morbidity and mortality rates for this age group, which is outside the range most often studied in terms of the morbidity and mortality paradox.

A final and important dimension affecting health-care access is the shortage of **bilingual** and **bicultural** health-care professionals. Carmen illustrates the problem of obtaining quality health care in Tucson, Arizona, for her Spanish-speaking mother:

> The quality of care, the attention, the miscommunication [that her mother experienced] . . . there were times in her life when she needed to see a counselor. No one in the city of Tucson could find a bilingual counselor. And I know for a fact that there are bilingual counselors, but the doctors had no idea where to look. That's almost a crime to me because there is a whole population that is not getting proper health care. . . . I really think something needs to be done, especially in the Southwest, where the Spanish-speaking population is growing so rapidly, and it has been so predominant for so many years. (Carmen G., 49)

To develop culturally competent interventions and increase the availability of culturally sensitive sites of care, there must be an adequate pool of Mexican-origin physicians and other health-care professionals. The current data illustrate that the percentage of health-care professionals who are of Mexican descent is disproportionately small compared to the size of this group. However, programs have been started to address this problem. The UC PRIME program, created by the University of California medical schools, tries to develop culturally competent health-care providers who can serve California's diverse community. This program may especially help Latinos, since California has a large proportion of Latinos.

Chapter 5 discusses the importance of cultural values and **linguistic competency** in ensuring quality health care for the Mexican-origin population. Linguistic competency is defined as the availability of health-care information in the language of the patient and the ability to communicate with patients in order to improve their health care. Providing linguistically competent care calls for added bilingual health-care providers and professionals. However, linguistic competency means more than translation or interpreter services. Linguistic competency is the first step in providing culturally competent care that meets the cultural needs of Spanish-speaking populations. A major factor to consider in providing linguistically and culturally competent health-care services is Mexican folklore. Many of the illnesses perceived as diseases in the Mexican-origin community are rooted in the spiritual and folkloric domains of Mexican culture. Folkloric illnesses may be treated with herbal remedies and spiritual practices such as *limpias* (ritual cleansings). These traditional remedies may either delay medical treatment of potentially serious illnesses or may complement medical treatment. Carmen's personal experience with folkloric remedies is described in the following vignette:

There were always some *hierbas* (herbs) not far away. Herbs and home remedies have been part of my upbringing, so I believe in them a lot. . . . I've always tried acupuncture and energy healing and that sort of thing. And I'm a firm believer that they do work because they worked for me. (Carmen G., 49)

Health-care professionals must be aware of culturally specific folkloric practices and beliefs, as well as the use of alternative treatments, such as folk remedies, which may influence diagnosis and treatment of an illness. Widespread use of alternative treatments within the Mexican-origin population may be limited; however, cultural practices of health and healing are prevalent in documented narratives of Latino health. Ethnic, gender, regional, and class differences within the Mexican-origin community play important roles in defining ethnic and cultural identity, which in turn affects perceptions of disease and appropriate treatment. Therefore, to serve this population well, health-care providers must be aware of these differences and cultural practices, as well as the degree of acculturation and biculturalism within the group they serve.

Medical personnel and staff can learn Spanish and achieve a measurable degree of linguistic competency, but achieving cultural competency is more complex. In general, the best bridge between the Mexican-origin population and the health-care system is through Mexican-origin health-care professionals. This group, by virtue of life experience, should be the most culturally competent. María expresses her preference for Latino health-care professionals this way:

If I were to need a therapist for psychological reasons, I would prefer to have a Hispanic because they would understand me a heck of a lot better than any Anglo would. A lot of the issues that we Hispanics have Anglos do not understand because of the culture. . . . I felt extremely comfortable with Dr. Duarte. . . . He was a Mexican, and there was a total comfort level with this doctor. . . . Somehow in my mind, I just felt that he understood. He understood where I was coming from, whatever issue it was, he seemed to be more sympathetic, he listened more, and was an excellent doctor. (María L., 44)

The unfortunate fact is that there are relatively few health-care professionals of Mexican descent. Thus, it is incumbent on us to pursue a dual strategy of educating all health-care professionals in the area of cultural competency while increasing the pool of qualified Latino health-care professionals. As the Mexican-origin population in the Southwest and other parts of the country continues to grow, improving its health and access to health care is vital to the overall health of the nation.

Chapter 6 concludes with a review of emergent issues that must be addressed if Mexican Americans and other Latino subgroups are to realize full participation in the U.S. health-care system.

Interviewee Personal Profiles

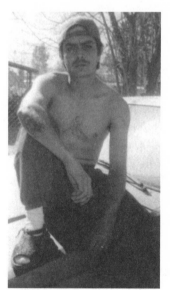

The following people were interviewed in the course of this book's preparation, to incorporate a sense of the everyday experiences of Mexicans and Mexican Americans in the U.S. health-care system. All interviewees are of Mexican origin.

Enrique Acuña Joy is a Mexicano who was born in Hermosillo, Sonora, Mexico. When he was interviewed in 2001, he was thirty years old and a restaurant worker in Arizona.

At the time of publication of this book's first edition, Lorena Bojórquez, a Latina from Nogales, Sonora, Mexico, was forty-eight years old and a homemaker.

Figure 2. Enrique Acuña.

Susie Duarte, a Mexican American woman born in San Diego, California, was forty years old and a self-employed child-care provider at the time of the interview in 2001. She obtained a degree from Santa Barbara City College.

Danny Flores (not his real name), a Mexican American born in California, was thirty-six years old when he was interviewed for this book's first edition. He was a coordinator for an agency that provides services for at-risk teenagers.

Marco Gámez of Agua Prieta, Sonora, graduated from the University of Arizona in December 1999 with a major in Mexican American studies and planned to attend law school. When the interview was conducted in 2001, Marco was twenty-eight years old and residing in Tucson, Arizona. He had recently received his U.S. citizenship.

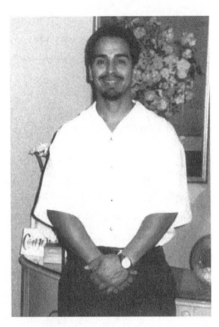

Figure 3. Marco Gámez.

At the time of the interview in 2001, Martín Fabián Gámez was thirty-one years old and employed by Motorola. He was born in Agua Prieta, Sonora, Mexico.

When interviewed for the first edition of this book, Francisco García, a Mexican American physician, was thirty-five years old and an

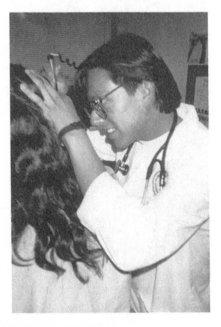

Figure 4. Dr. Francisco García.

assistant professor of obstetrics and gynecology at University Medical Center in Tucson, Arizona. His research focused on cervical cancer screening along the U.S.-Mexico border.

Carmen Gastelum is a Chicana from Nogales, Arizona, who worked in Colorado as a financial services consultant. When interviewed for the first edition of this book, she was forty-nine years old and a resident of Tucson, Arizona.

María Lobato, who was forty-four years old when interviewed for the first edition of this book, is a Mexicana from Tijuana, Mexico. She was a case manager for dental and optical services at the St. Elizabeth of Hungary Clinic in Arizona.

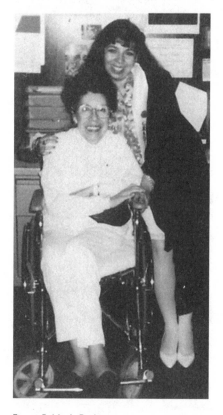

Figure 5. María Pacho.

At the time of the 2001 interview, Ana Manzano was twenty-six years old and a bilingual second-grade teacher. She was born in Tucson, Arizona.

During the initial interview for the first edition of this book, Yolanda Nielba, a Mexican American woman born in Guadalajara, Jalisco, Mexico, was fifty-two years old. She was an operator for Data Corporation.

María Pacho, a Latina from East Los Angeles, California, was thirty-one years old at the time of the interview in 2001. She was the supervisor of the Youth Opportunity Movement program in the Los Angeles Community Development Department. Pacho has a master's degree in public health from

Loma Linda University and received a bachelor's degree in Chicano/ Latino studies from Cal State Long Beach.

Ernie Pérez, a Mexican American man, is a fourth generation Tucsonan. At the time of the initial interview in 2001, he was forty years old and the program manager for Salud y El Poder: The Latino Men's Health Project, which provided health education services to residents of Tucson and Sonora.

Lily Quiñones, a Latino college student from El Paso, Texas, was twenty years old at the time of the interview in 2001. She was majoring in family studies at the University of Arizona.

When the interview took place in 2001, Marissia Quiroga, a Mexican American, was twenty-two years old and a nursing student at Santa Barbara City College. She was a part-time employee at St. Francis Hospital in Santa Barbara. She expected to graduate in the fall of 1999 and planned to pursue her bachelor's degree.

When interviewed for the first edition of this book, Refugio Rochín, a Mexican American from Colton, California, was fifty-seven years old. He holds a PhD in agricultural economics and was the director of the Smithsonian Center for Latino Initiatives, which is part of the Smithsonian Institution in Washington, DC.

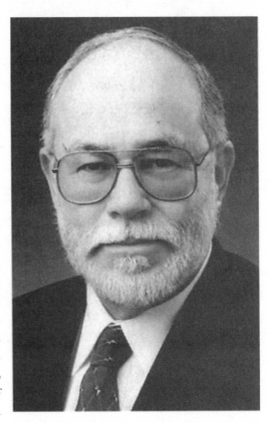

Figure 6. Dr. Refugio Rochín.

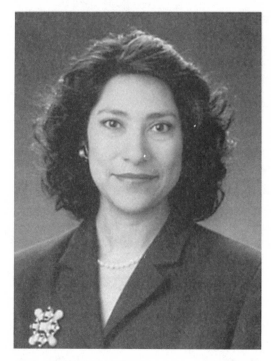

When the initial interview took place in 2001, Graciela (Gracie) Guzmán Saenz was forty-six years old and working as a lawyer specializing in international law and business transactions. Born and raised in Houston, Texas, Saenz was the first Mexican American woman to run for mayor of that city; she was also a former member of the Houston City Council.

Figure 7. Graciela Guzmán Saenz.

Notes

1. After Proposition 187 and the changes in the federal welfare reform bill of 1996, a significant discussion ensued in Congress about limiting the right of legal immigrants to access health-care programs such as Medicaid. The purpose of limiting such access was to discourage the legalization of low-income immigrants.

2. Either the woman or her husband must pay into the fund for forty quarters to be eligible for Medicare.

Chapter 1

An Introduction to the Mexican-Origin Population

"It Was Just an Ideal Location"

My parents developed their business in community relations around provisions and Mexican food and supplies for small Mexican businesses. From the start, they instilled upon me the value of hard work, the value of being Mexican, providing products and services for the Mexican community. They also instilled upon me the importance of family. I cannot say my family ever hindered me. On the contrary, my family looks towards me as being special, encouraged me, and supported me in all activities I undertook, even though at times they didn't know what I was doing. Anytime I spoke to them, they always thought I was doing something new, different, and great. They were always very supportive. (Refugio R., 57)

My parents were always hard-working people. My father taught me work ethic. He was an individual that believed in work, and his philosophy of life [was], "If you work, you don't starve. No matter how poor you may be, a good day's work you can do." He expected us to be up bright and early, and to be working constantly, and that's been my lifestyle ever since. (Gracie S., 46)

Refugio Rochín and Graciela Saenz represent both the diversity and strong work ethic that characterize many Mexican Americans in the United States. They are members of the country's largest Latino subgroup, and their roots are in the Southwest. One is the son of native-born Mexican Americans, the other the daughter of Mexican immigrants. Even though they share similar cultural backgrounds, they have their own unique histories. This convergence of cultural traits, individual identity, and common history forms the complex tapestry that is the Mexican American experience.

In this chapter, we will examine how individual health is intricately related to environmental and sociodemographic conditions. Because factors such as age, education, immigrant status, and occupation, as well as genetic factors, influence the risk of specific health problems, we will provide an overview of the variables (measurable elements) that affect the health status of the Mexican-origin population. These variables must be understood within the historical experience of this group in the United States. By framing these factors within their political, geographic, historic, and economic context, we enhance our understanding of health problems affecting Mexican Americans and increase our chances of finding solutions to them. For example, the historical concentration of the Mexican-origin population in the nation's southern border region explains the current political-geographic location of the bulk of this group in the Southwest. We have divided this chapter into seven sections: political-geographic concentration, historical factors influencing population growth and location, language status, Human Development Index, educational level, occupational location, and concluding thoughts.

Political-Geographic Concentration of the Mexican-Origin Population

A major factor affecting the health status of Mexican Americans is where they live. The fact that they are concentrated in the Southwest results in regional influences that affect both the delivery and quality of health care. For example, Mexican Americans who live in the border region have a different quality of health care than those in urban areas such as Chicago. While inequalities may exist in both locations, different political and institutional environments affect the health-care systems in various states and regions. Another important factor is whether Mexican Americans are a significant percentage of both the general and Latino population of a state or region, as this too will set the cultural context in which we recommend health policies.

The Mexican-origin population makes up more than 64 percent of the entire Latino population of the United States. Almost 72 percent of Mexican-descent individuals reside in the southwestern states of Arizona, California, Colorado, New Mexico, and Texas—with California and Texas accounting for 62 percent of the total. Recent data shows, however, that the fastest Latino growth rates are in unlikely places such as South Carolina, Tennessee, and North Carolina. Midwestern **metropolitan areas** such as Chicago have long had significant Mexican-origin populations as well.

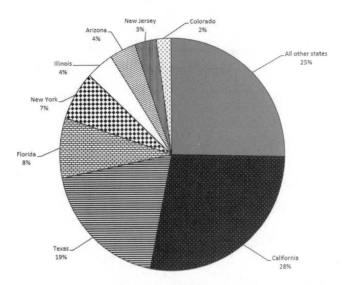

Figure 8. U.S. Census Bureau percent distribution of the Hispanic/Latino population by state in 2010. Source: U.S. Census Bureau, 2010, *Census Summary File 1*. http://www.census.gov/.

Thus, the growth of this Latino subpopulation within the last twenty years has been rapid and has reached beyond the Southwest.

The current growth of the Mexican-origin population relative to the **non-Latino** population in the Southwest can be attributed to two major factors: (1) a higher **fertility rate** in the Mexican-origin population, and (2) immigration. Figure 8 illustrates the size of the Mexican-origin population by state in 2010.

Table 1 shows the percentage of Mexican-origin people within each of the southwestern states relative to that state's overall Latino population based on the U.S. Census Bureau's American Community Survey in 2012. The three states with the largest concentration of Mexican-origin Latinos relative to other Latino subpopulations are Arizona, California, and Texas. People of Mexican origin represent more than 80 percent of the total Latino population of these three states. Since the southern borders of Texas and Arizona alone account for more than 1,600 miles of the U.S.-Mexico border, it is not surprising that they contain significant points of entry for documented and undocumented Mexicans coming into the United States.

The concentration of Mexican Americans in the southwest border region has unique health implications. First, the rapid population growth on both sides of the U.S.-Mexico border has placed great pressure on the limited

Table 1.   Mexican Americans as a Percentage of the Total Latino Population in Five Southwestern States

STATE	TOTAL LATINO POPULATION IN STATE	PERCENTAGE OF MEXICAN ORIGIN
Arizona	1,976,104	90.1
California	14,537,661	83.3
Colorado	1,088,742	75.0
New Mexico	979,724	62.7
Texas	9,960,910	87.7

Source: American Community Survey, B03001: Selected Population Profile in the United States, in *2012 American Community Survey 1-Year Estimates.*

public health infrastructure of this area. As a result border residents are at greater risk of exposure to infectious diseases as well as environmental hazards. Second, both the U.S. border population and the Mexican border population are politically isolated from their respective federal governments. Therefore, they have limited ability to influence the reallocation of government resources to the border region. Thus, health issues may be ignored or health services may be underfunded until a catastrophic health event occurs.

California has the largest number of Mexican-origin people, with more than twelve million. Many of the Mexican-origin residents of California are newcomers, as California, like New York, is a magnet for various immigrant groups. This is partly due to California's rich employment base, ethnic enclaves that provide kinship relationships to recent immigrants, and relatively generous public infrastructure that assists immigrants in integrating into mainstream American society. In addition to the large Mexican-origin population in California, other Latino groups, such as Guatemalans and Salvadorans, are well represented. These groups are located within, or in close proximity to, Mexican-origin communities. More than 60 percent of California's Latino population resides in just five of its fifty-eight counties: Los Angeles County, Orange County, San Bernardino County, Riverside County, and San Diego County. These southern counties, which stretch from the Mexican border north to Los Angeles, reflect the uneven concentration of the Mexican-origin population within the state.

Colorado and New Mexico also have relatively large Mexican-origin populations. New Mexico, however, is uniquely characterized by its sizable

Hispano/a population, with deep roots that well precede statehood and, in some instances, are linked to Spanish colonial times.[1] Thus, many New Mexicans define their identity more as Hispano/a or Nuevo Mexicanos than as Mexican Americans. Although the case of Hispanos/as in New Mexico is interesting, they represent a small proportion of the total U.S. Mexican-origin population.

In California and Texas the Mexican-origin figure reaches almost one in three. In Arizona, more than one in four residents is of Mexican origin. In New Mexico, the Hispano/Mexican-origin ratio is almost one in two. Underlying the present immigration and fertility trends are many historical factors that have influenced the geographic concentration of this group in the Southwest. The proximity of the U.S.-Mexico border provided an entry point for earlier immigrants and continues to be an entry point for more recent ones. Yet the historical legacy of Spanish and Mexican settlement patterns predates current national boundaries. Spain, and later Mexico, had control of this area for more than a century before it was lost to the United States. This early history is the initial basis for the settlement patterns of the Mexican-origin population.

Another important trend is the rapid growth of the **foreign-born** Mexican-origin population, particularly in California (see table 2). This can be attributed to the significance of Mexico as an immigrant-sending country. It is also a result of the Immigration Reform and Control Act (IRCA), which allowed immigrants who had lived continuously in the United States without legal documentation since before January 1, 1982, to legalize their status between the time of the law's passage in 1986 and May 4, 1988. As the vast majority of these immigrants were of Mexican origin, IRCA disproportionately affected the status of Mexican immigrants.

Table 2. Foreign-Born versus Native-Born Mexican-Origin Population in Five Southwestern States, 2009

STATE	NATIVE-BORN (%)	FOREIGN-BORN (%)
Arizona	69	31
California	63	37
Colorado	70	30
New Mexico	76	24
Texas	70	30

Source: American Community Survey, S0201: Selected Population Profile in the United States, in *2009 American Community Survey 1-Year Estimates.*

The majority of immigrants legalized during this period resided in two states: California and Texas. This further increased the capacity of ethnic enclaves to establish support systems for future Mexican immigrants with similar Mexican community roots. Thus, these communities became an easier entrance point for foreign-born immigrants, which helps explain the differential concentration of foreign-born immigrants in the Southwest.

Historical Concentration of the Mexican-Origin Population

The roots and kinship ties that were established when the U.S. Southwest was part of Mexico are the basis for the disproportionate concentration of Mexican-origin people there. Much of what is now known as the American Southwest was Spanish territory (New Spain) for three centuries prior to Mexican independence in 1821. After Mexico became an independent nation, a significant segment of its territory was in the path of a rapidly expanding United States. A key turning point in the history of the U.S.-Mexico borderlands took place in 1848. This date marks the end of the brief but bitter U.S.-Mexican War, which drastically altered the geographic boundaries of both countries. As a result of this war, Mexico lost a significant portion of its territory, which had included the present-day U.S. states of California, Arizona, New Mexico, Texas, Utah, Nevada, and parts of Colorado, Wyoming, Oklahoma, and Kansas. In 1853, the **Gadsden Purchase** changed the boundary again to include within the United States additional portions of present-day New Mexico and Arizona. The year 1848 also marks the important **Treaty of Guadalupe Hidalgo**, which ended the U.S.-Mexican War. It defined, among other points, the property and civil rights of the Mexican and Hispano/a population in the territory ceded by Mexico to the United States.[2] The following maps (figures 9 through 12) illustrate the shifting political boundaries of the American Southwest and show how, despite U.S. westward expansion, Hispano/Mexican roots remained deeply embedded in the political, social, and historical traditions linked to Mexican and Spanish culture.[3]

The deep cultural roots are linked to the political-geographical settlement patterns of many Mexican Americans, as illustrated by the experience of Carmen Gastelum:

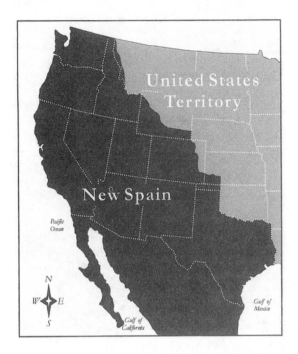

Figure 9. Border between New Spain and the United States, 1800–1819.

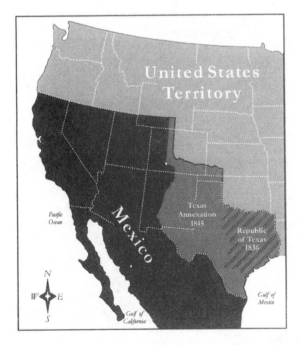

Figure 10. Border between Mexico and the United States, 1819–1848.

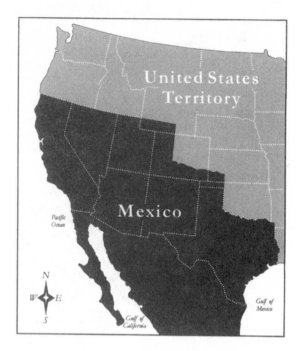

Figure 11. Border between Mexico and the United States, 1821.

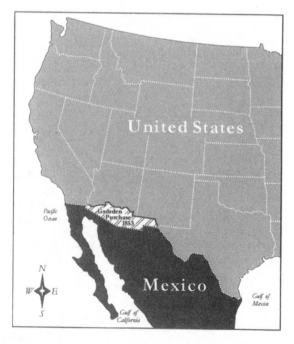

Figure 12. Border between Mexico and the United States, 1848–present.

My mother's side of the family came from Sonora—Hermosillo—and my father's family came across on a French ship. They mixed up with the Seri Indians and came north with the Yaqui Indians until they came up to Arizona before it was the U.S., and settled in the Santa Cruz Valley.

Knowing the history of the Mexican-origin population, particularly in the Southwest, is important because it helps us understand current migration flows and ethnic concentrations. This knowledge also helps put into context the current tensions within the Mexican-origin community over land rights, identity, and marginalization from the power structures of American society. In addition to recognizing landownership, the Treaty of Guadalupe Hidalgo guaranteed that individuals who lived within the Mexican territory ceded to the United States would be given full political rights as U.S. citizens and that their civil rights would be protected. Unfortunately, U.S. federal and state governments failed to honor and comply with the treaty's requirements after the war, reflecting the escalating negative sentiments toward Mexicans that further fueled ethnic and racial divisions within the Southwest.[4] These historical and political factors influence how and when Mexican Americans enter the health-care system and how they are treated within it.

Given this historical context we can begin to understand the pervasiveness of conflict between the dominant non-Latino power structure and the Mexican-origin population over land, language, and equity issues. Notwithstanding this conflict, Mexican settlement in the southern border region continues. Today, growth in border regions and ethnic enclaves of the Southwest affects both the Mexican-origin and larger non-Latino communities. According to historian Oscar Martínez, the borderland milieu has enormous implications for a nation. "The expansion of economic activity in a border zone means population growth at the margin of the nation and consequent migration ... across the boundary. Finally, questions of national identity emerge as borderlanders fuse their culture with that of their neighbors, creating new social patterns that people in the heartland zones may find abhorrent."[5] Thus, new tension points emerge as Mexican nationals increasingly migrate beyond the border, influencing both the cultural and sociodemographic composition of American society. These tensions are exacerbated by the resiliency and growth of the Spanish language in the border region as well as in large cities such as Los Angeles and Houston, where recent Mexican immigrants have become the dominant group. Such population growth and cultural shift in the urban core of the Southwest has created growing concern over how health-care resources should be delivered and used.

Language Status

> Well, actually I'm bilingual, so it's been great. If I wasn't bilingual, there would definitely be a problem. . . . I'm talking in Spanish and English [at work]. . . . You definitely need to be bilingual. (María L., 44)

Many of the central issues of Mexican-origin identity and economic status within the broader U.S. society are framed within the context of the Spanish language. Today many health-care professionals realize that Spanish language fluency is a critical skill for providing quality service to the Mexican-origin population. Language constitutes a symbolic component of ethnic identity for many members of this group. Spanish is inextricably linked to Mexican identity, and often it is difficult to separate the two. Thus occurs what Margarita Hidalgo identifies as the "Spanish Mexican equation," which highlights an interesting contradiction: the Spanish language is sometimes viewed as an asset and sometimes as a liability. In the former case, Spanish links the individual to the home culture, and in the latter case it excludes the individual from mainstream U.S. society.[6] The Mexican-origin community often experiences an internal conflict that manifests itself in the struggle to maintain the Spanish language while striving for economic assimilation into American society. In most instances, economic assimilation requires English skills and fluency, yet this fluency may result in a loss of the familial language. For some Mexican Americans this loss is viewed as a betrayal of one's own ethnic roots, given the historical context in which Mexicans were punished socially and economically for speaking Spanish. At the same time, many Mexican-origin families who live outside the border region have less exposure to Spanish-speaking recent immigrants. For them the decline of Spanish language use and eventual language loss may occur naturally through the process of intergenerational change and assimilation into U.S. society. This division between cultural assimilation and intergenerational progress, given the historical reality of language and cultural discrimination, has created for many a need to symbolically resist cultural and language immersion and retain the Spanish language and cultural beliefs as an essential part of one's Mexican identity. This resistance in Mexican-origin communities throughout the Southwest has resulted in a backlash from a large segment of white non-Latino voters. This is best illustrated in the passage of **Arizona's HB 2281** in 2010, which banned Ethnic Studies, specifically Mexican American Studies, curricula in district-owned schools.

Many Mexican American leaders in the state lobbied against this initiative based on their fear that it was racially motivated, as it targeted primarily Spanish-speaking Mexican immigrants. Thus, this proposition galvanized the Spanish-speaking community for two reasons: because of a common ethnic identity that is heavily tied to cultural and language identity and because of continued concern over institutionalized discrimination by the state.

There is now evidence of a reverse language shift in some Mexican ethnic enclaves, particularly in the border region. Reverse language shift occurs when Spanish supersedes English as the dominant language.[7] Unfortunately, this does not occur without a backlash from some members of the dominant society, who view widespread Spanish use as "un-American." An excellent example of this backlash occurred when the city council of the Texas border town of El Cenizo decided to conduct its monthly meetings in Spanish. This decision was aimed at providing greater access to the government for the citizens, most of whom speak Spanish. In fact, Spanish is the dominant language in El Cenizo. This local decision created a national uproar that was fomented by talk show hosts and nativist groups opposed to bilingualism. The following excerpt from nationally syndicated radio talk show hosts Don Geronimo and Mike O'Meara during an on-air interview with one of El Cenizo's town commissioners, Flora Barton, illustrates the hostility.

Barton: We speak Spanish to the people that do not understand English.

Don: Get on your burro and go back to Mayheeco! . . . If those people do not understand my language, they should get on their burros and go back to Mayheeco.

Barton: You have to understand that if someone speaks Spanish, that does not make them un-American or any less of an American.

Don: You people have your own country. Why are you trying to ruin our language?[8]

The reaction to the language policy of El Cenizo graphically illustrates the existing racism toward Mexican-origin people. In this case, Spanish is symbolic of the perceived threat that Mexican culture poses to the dominant way of life. On the other hand, El Cenizo town leaders recognize that to effectively deliver public services such as health care, the dominant town language, Spanish, has to be used.

In spite of the white backlash originating in nonborder areas of the United States, the Spanish language has resiliency because of the continual influx of Mexican immigrants. Moreover, many health-care systems in the region are now requiring their providers to have some degree of fluency in Spanish. In the Southwest, significant portions of the Mexican American population may be characterized as bilingual. As illustrated in table 3, with the exception of Colorado and New Mexico, more than 70 percent of all Mexican-origin individuals are bilingual. Moreover, in the two largest southwestern states, approximately 35 percent of the Mexican-origin population does not speak English well. Thus, for a major portion of the Mexican-origin population in the Southwest, language fluency will continue to be an important issue.

Social science research indicates that, beyond the historical and symbolic dimensions of a language, fluency in English is a key to educational and economic mobility in the United States. An extensive body of literature indicates that English language skills and proficiency play an important role in the educational and economic success of Mexican-origin people. Moreover, subtle differences in language fluency such as grammatical skills, accented English, and conversational fluency are important predictors of income and socioeconomic status for Mexican-origin persons in the United States.[9] Without English fluency, educational attainment is severely constrained and prospects

Table 3.   English Language Ability of Mexican-Origin People in Five Southwestern States (Five Years of Age or Older)

STATE	SPEAK LANGUAGE OTHER THAN ENGLISH (%)	DO NOT SPEAK ENGLISH "VERY WELL" (%)
Arizona	70.3	30.2
California	77.5	37.5
Colorado	60.2	31.5
New Mexico	67.1	25.3
Texas	78.4	34.4

Source: American Community Survey, S0201: Selected Population Profile in the United States, in 2009 American Community Survey 1-Year Estimates.

for economic mobility are limited. Lack of fluency also impedes effective communication in the sphere of social services such as health care. The significance of the latter point is illustrated by Jill Reichman's study, in which she states that for many Mexican Americans, regardless of English ability, Spanish is the native language and therefore the "language of illness and somatic [bodily] distress."[10] Thus, the issue of language use includes a practical component that affects the employment and health status of many people.

Human Development Index

The American Human Development Index (a modified version of the global Human Development Index) is a project undertaken by the Social Sciences Research Council as part of their Measure of America program. Traditionally, the well-being of a country, and therefore its people, is captured by economic indicators such as Gross National Product (GNP) or per capita GNP. The Human Development Index uses the progress and opportunities available to people, rather than a country or state's economy, to measure the progress and well-being of the people.

The American Human Development Index is a combination of multiple factors of human development that result in a number from 0 to 10. This number can be used to compare the well-being and development of different subpopulations and geographic regions. Three main factors are used to evaluate the well-being of a country, region, or state: health, education, and income. Overall, the United States has a Human Development Index of 5.03 when these different factors are all taken into consideration. Comparatively, Latinos have a Human Development Index of 4.05. But what does that mean? The next few paragraphs describe the particular measurements of the Human Development Index and how Latinos compare to the United States population as a whole.

The American Human Development Index uses life expectancy as the measure of health for different states, ethnic groups, and genders. The prospect of a healthy, lasting life is universally important for quality of life. Latinos as a group have the second highest life expectancy of any ethnic group in America. Latinos are expected to live, on average, 82.8 years (compared to the national average of 78.9 years). When gender is taken into account, Latina women live the second longest after Asian American women, and Latino men are in the middle compared to other ethnic groups and genders.

Education is used as a measurement component of human development because education provides "access to knowledge," which allows people to make decisions about their lives. Overall, Latinos have the lowest level of educational attainment of any ethnic group. Only 13.0 percent of Latinos have a Bachelor's degree, compared to the national average of 28.2 percent, and only 4.1 percent of Latinos have any type of graduate degree, compared to the national average of 10.4 percent. Additionally, 37.8 percent of Latinos have less than a high school level of education, a significantly higher percentage than the national rate of 14.4 percent. When gender is taken into account, Latino men have the lowest levels of educational attainment of any racial/ethnic group. Latina women have the third lowest level of attainment, despite the fact that women have higher rates of educational attainment than men.

Income, which the American Human Development Index describes as a "decent standard of living," is defined as the middle level of personal income a person earns in a year. In 2010 dollars, Latinos were the lowest earners of any other ethnic/racial group, with an average personal income of $20,956. That amount is almost $8,000 less than the average income for the United States as a whole. Latina women are the lowest earners of either gender of any ethnicity/racial group. Latino men ranked somewhere in the middle, just under white women. Even though women in general had a higher level of education attainment then men, men as a whole still out-earned women.

Latinos are right in the middle compared to other ethnic groups in terms of their overall American Human Development Index of 4.05. Even though Latinos generally have lower levels of education and income compared to

Table 4. Human Development Index Indicators Based on Subpopulations

	HUMAN DEVELOPMENT INDEX	LIFE EXPECTANCY	BACHELOR'S DEGREE	AVERAGE INDIVIDUAL INCOME
United States (as a whole)	5.03	78.9 years	28.2%	$28,899
Asian Americans	7.21	86.5 years	50.2%	$34,415
Whites	5.43	78.9 years	31.4%	$31,681
Latinos	4.05	82.8 years	13.0%	$20,956
African Americans	3.81	74.6 years	17.9%	$24,974
Native Americans	3.55	76.9 years	14.2%	$21,863

Source: Sarah Burd-Sharps and Kristen Lewis, American Human Development Report: The Measure of America, 2013–2014.

other groups, the long life expectancy of Latinos plays a pivotal role in their overall well-being. The relatively good health status of Latinos, regardless of their ability to pay for health care or their educational levels, is a concept that we will discuss in later chapters.

Educational Level

> To me, education is so important because it will make me a better person. I am going to learn something that I will be able to use for the rest of my life. Not only that, it's going to help me make decisions that will help me to succeed and make more money to [be] financially set when I [am] at an age where I can no longer work. (Martín G., 31)

> When I was growing up my father always used to say that we could graduate, as girls we could graduate up to high school, but afterwards he expected us to work and contribute to the family. To him, there was no need for me to go to college, 'cause I would probably just get married, have kids, and there would be no need for it. And so his understanding of the role of the woman was very difficult or very different from what was actually taking place in the U.S. My father had actually been raised in Mexico and came to the U.S. as an adult, so his understanding of the role of [women], how he thought he should raise us as women was a conflict in my life, and a real struggle. (Gracie S., 46)

Educational attainment is another important factor influencing the health status of the Mexican-origin population. Level of education influences the occupational status of Mexican-origin people in all parts of the United States; occupational status in turn predicts whether or not they will rely on public or private health-care services. Education also influences the extent to which individuals are aware of risky behaviors or of predisposing conditions that may influence their own health. For example, in states such as California, Colorado, and Texas, where there are large Mexican immigrant populations, more than 40 percent of the Mexican-origin population twenty-five years and older has less than a high school diploma. In the other southwestern border states, with the exception of Arizona and New Mexico, less than 60 percent of the Mexican-origin population within this category has a high school diploma. Furthermore, with the exception of Colorado and New Mexico, less than 10 percent of the Mexican-origin population twenty-five years or older have a baccalaureate degree (see figure

13). Education status among this group is a hotly debated issue because of three observable trends. First, the Mexican-origin population has one of the highest high school dropout rates and one of the lowest college completion rates in the nation. Second, educational policies such as bilingual and English as a Second Language (ESL) education—which were created to improve educational attainment and rectify past discrimination against language-minority students—are under public scrutiny and attack. Third, given the increasingly globalized and high-skill-based U.S. economy, continued poor academic performance may result in further socioeconomic segregation.

The failure of America's public schools to educate the Mexican-origin population adequately is rooted in segregation. Institutionalized, or **de jure**, segregation of this group in southwestern schools occurred between 1900 and 1950, and **de facto segregation** still occurs.[11] In light of the educational discrimination against the Mexican-origin population in the Southwest, community leaders developed educational policies and programs to address both linguistic and cultural differences. The first of these programs was bilingual education, which was enacted into law in 1968 during the Nixon administration with the passing of the Bilingual Education Act.

The importance of bilingual education cannot be overstated; it was the first attempt to rectify systematic discrimination in the public schools

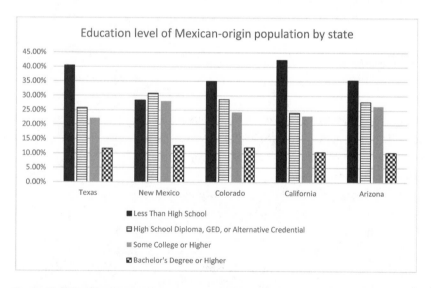

Figure 13. Educational level of the Mexican-origin population, by state (ages twenty-five and older). Source: American Community Survey, S0201: Selected Population Profile in the United States, in *2010 American Community Survey 1-Year Estimates*.

against the Mexican-origin population based on linguistic differences. These programs have been successful in addressing linguistic discrimination, but issues of adequate funding and implementation plagued them. Although bilingual education was critical in rectifying past educational discrimination, the shift in the demographic profile has limited the implementation and success of these programs, as well as the adverse impact from white non-Latino voter backlash. With the decline of the original bilingual language education programs, English as a Second Language (ESL) programs increasingly focused on English-language acquisition skills with a more measured English language learning program approach that would accelerate English language acquisition.

In reality, bilingual education and ESL programs alone cannot address the complexity of educational issues facing Mexican Americans. Individual characteristics, such as immigration status, as well as household characteristics, such as parental education and poverty levels, are important predictors of educational success in addition to the environmental factors that directly impact schools. These factors further complicate the use of specific strategies such as bilingual education and ESL in addressing educational attainment problems. Future education policies will need to address these surrounding factors if they are to be successful.

Occupational Location

Educational attainment is directly linked to **occupational location**, which refers to the type of job and economic sector in which a person is employed. Therefore, educational attainment and educational policy ultimately have critical implications for the economic success of Mexican Americans. For example, Mexican Americans who are employed in low-tier jobs such as farm labor are at greater risk for job-related injuries such as pesticide poisoning.

Overall, the distribution of Mexican Americans in the U.S. economy is largely concentrated in lower-tier blue-collar and service employment. In the Southwest, the Mexican-origin population is still employed in low-income occupations. For example, in Arizona, almost half of Mexican-origin workers are employed in agriculture, construction, and service jobs. In California, a state that is heavily dependent on agricultural production, while less than 5 percent of the Mexican-origin population is employed in agriculture, over 40 percent is employed in the agriculture, construction, and service sectors combined (see figures 14 through 18). Racial discrimination also influences the employment of many Mexicans within the Southwest. Perhaps no sector in the U.S. economy captures this historical reality as profoundly as the agricultural sector, due to three main factors: (1) the early dominance of agricultural interests in developing this labor market; (2) the recurring shortage of low-skilled labor in this sector, given the wages and working conditions; and (3) the ideological need of federal and state officials to racialize labor market policies to justify unequal wage and working conditions for fieldworkers. The last point is important as historically it allowed for the exclusion of agricultural workers from key legislation influencing the degree of collective bargaining in this market. This prevented farmworkers from unionizing sooner, which also limited their access to health insurance. In addition, immigration policy was flexible with respect to migrant seasonal workers, allowing for a continuous flow of low-wage Mexican labor to the agricultural fields of the Southwest. Such policies contributed to a racialized labor market in the region, which further limited the political participation of Mexican immigrants in the debates over national and state health policy.

Racialized labor markets systematically placed Mexican-origin workers in specific segments of employment and wage categories. This practice was common in the major sectors that employed Mexican workers for most of

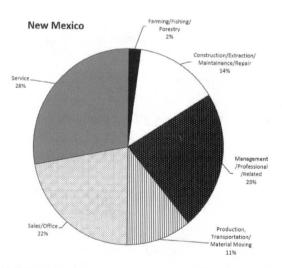

Figure 14. Occupations of Mexican-origin people: New Mexico. Source: American Community Survey, S0201: Selected Population Profile in the United States, in *2009 American Community Survey 1-year Estimates.*

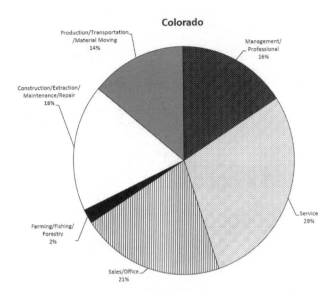

Figure 15. Occupations of Mexican-origin people: Colorado. Source: American Community Survey, S0201: Selected Population Profile in the United States, in *2009 American Community Survey 1-Year Estimates*.

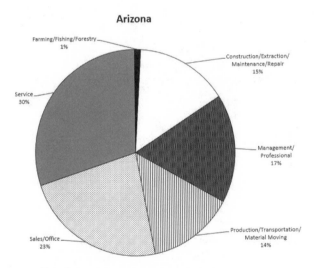

Figure 16. Occupations of Mexican-origin people: Arizona. Source: American Community Survey, S0201: Selected Population Profile in the United States, in *2009 American Community Survey 1-Year Estimates*.

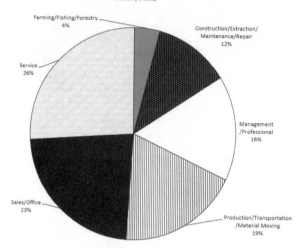

California

Farming/Fishing/Forestry
4%

Construction/Extraction/
Maintenance/Repair
12%

Service
26%

Management
/Professional
16%

Sales/Office
23%

Production/Transportation
/Material Moving
19%

Figure 17. Occupations of Mexican-origin people: California. Source: American Community Survey, S0201: Selected Population Profile in the United States, in *2009 American Community Survey 1-Year Estimates.*

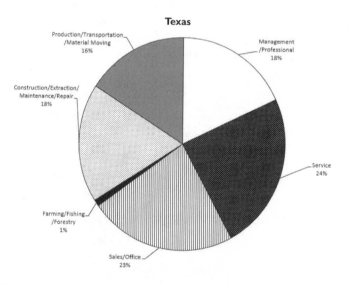

Texas

Production/Transportation
/Material Moving
16%

Management
/Professional
18%

Construction/Extraction/
Maintenance/Repair
18%

Service
24%

Farming/Fishing
/Forestry
1%

Sales/Office
23%

Figure 18. Occupations of Mexican-origin people: Texas. Source: American Community Survey, S0201: Selected Population Profile in the United States, in *2009 American Community Survey 1-Year Estimates.*

the twentieth century, such as agriculture, ranching, mining, railroads, and the industrial blue-collar and service industries. As scholar Mario Barrera has noted, "Occupational stratification remained an even more marked characteristic of the urban labor system in the first three decades of the century, as data for several major cities make clear."[12]

Many farmworkers still have no means of obtaining quality health care or related services, even though they face disproportionate exposure to work-related health hazards such as direct contact with pesticides and other toxic chemicals that cause illness or even death. The mainstream environmental movement had recognized the danger of pesticide exposure as a valid concern by 1960. However, it was not until 1965 that the plight of farmworkers, especially those in California, finally received widespread attention with the help of farm labor activist César Chávez. Between 1965 and 1971, the campaign for farmworkers' rights, fair wages, and better living conditions also challenged health and environmentally related civil rights violations such as pesticide exposure.[13]

Exposure to pesticides is just one of the many occupational health hazards that plague Mexican-origin workers. Their overrepresentation in blue-collar and manual-labor jobs places them at higher risk for exposure to work hazards, which in turn affects their overall health status. Workers are often unaware that they have been or are being exposed to harmful materials, such as pesticides, and therefore do not report incidents to company superiors or health-care professionals. They rarely recognize that many chronic health problems and illnesses are work related or are caused by prolonged exposure to chemicals and an unsafe work environment.

Although agriculture is no longer the dominant sector for Mexican-origin workers, their continued employment in low-tier service and blue-collar jobs contributes to the creation of problems similar to those of the past. Further, because of their overrepresentation in low-wage jobs, many are isolated in poor ethnic enclaves (neighborhoods) where environmental hazards are also frequently present.

Figures 14 to 18 illustrate the dominant sectors of employment for Mexican-origin workers in five states of the Southwest. These charts highlight the occupational categories that influence the health status profile of this population. Notwithstanding the current debates on immigration restrictions, the demand for low-wage Mexican immigrant workers continues to relegate these workers to the lowest occupational segments of the U.S. economy. This has direct implications for the health of Mexican workers and that of their families. As is the case with agricultural workers, these lower-tiered jobs pose greater risks of work-related injuries, unsafe working conditions, and environmental hazards. Adding to the risk of such jobs is the fact that they are less likely to offer health insurance.

Concluding Thoughts

This chapter has highlighted the relationship between the political-geographic location of the Mexican-origin population and its present health status. Both have been influenced by the history of what is today the American Southwest. Discrimination and segregation in schools and the labor market have contributed to present-day inequalities in health care. The location of Mexican-origin communities is important because it influences language proficiency in English and Spanish, as well as educational and occupational opportunities, thus affecting the health of community members. In addition, social networks in established ethnic enclaves largely influence immigrant settlement patterns. These boundaries ultimately influence the cultural milieu of this group, its social and work environments, and its help-seeking patterns, including its access to health care.

This chapter also provides an overview of selected sociodemographic variables and environmental factors that influence the present-day health status of the Mexican-origin population. Among these variables are language, education, immigrant status, and occupation. In addition, it is possible to expand and refine these predictors by including variables such as marital status, family size, age, poverty status, and income level. These broad characteristics provide a basis for understanding the factors underlying health-care access, environmentally related health issues, and cultural and linguistic beliefs and behaviors. Genetic factors, which will be explored in the next chapter, also play an important role.

Discussion Exercises

1. What factors should be considered in defining the health status of the Mexican-origin population? What indicators can be used to measure health status?

2. How has the historical experience of Mexican Americans affected their geographic concentration, language use, and the formation of ethnic enclaves?

3. Discuss the links between variables such as language, education, and occupation and the socioeconomic status of the Mexican-origin population in the United States.

4. How has continuous Mexican immigration affected the overall status of the U.S. Mexican-origin population in terms of language, culture, education, and health status?

5. How has legislation directed toward the Mexican-origin population affected their legal status and access to education and health-care services?

6. How are Spanish language and ethnic identity connected? What are different ways in which these concepts are constructed and perceived within and outside the Mexican American community?

7. How does the concentration of Mexican-origin workers in certain sectors of the U.S. economy affect earnings, working conditions, and health risks?

Notes

1. S. Rodríguez, "The Hispano Homeland Debate Revisited," *Perspectives in Mexican American Studies* 3 (1992): 98. Inclusion of Hispanos/as in the Mexican American ethnic group is widely accepted, even by those who support this group's claim to cultural uniqueness. According to Rodríguez, "none of the principals seem seriously to be denying that Hispanos are Mexican Americans."

2. O. J. Martínez, *Border People* (Tucson: University of Arizona Press, 1994), 27–33.

3. The maps are compiled from the following sources: Martínez, *Border People*; L. M. Metz, *Border: The U.S.-Mexico Line* (El Paso, TX: Mangan Books, 1989); J. J. Wagoner, *Arizona: Its Place in the United States* (Salt Lake City: Peregrine Smith Books, 1989) and *Arizona's Heritage* (Salt Lake City: Peregrine Smith Books, 1987); and A. Wexler, *Atlas of Westward Expansion* (New York: Facts on File, 1995).

4. D. Gutiérrez, *Walls and Mirrors* (Berkeley: University of California Press, 1995), 17–18, 20.

5. Martínez, *Border People*, 25.

6. M. Hidalgo, "Language and Ethnicity in the 'Taboo' Region: The U.S.-Mexico Border," *International Journal of the Sociology of Language* 114 (1995): 31.

7. Ibid.

8. "Excerpts from Don and Mike's Messages of Hatred to Hispanics," *Hispanic Link Weekly Report* 17, no. 34 (August 30, 1999): 3.

9. See A. Dávila, A. K. Bohara, and R. Saenz, "Accent Penalties and the Earnings of Mexican Americans," *Social Science Quarterly* 74, no. 4 (December 1993): 902–15; or

K. E. Espinosa and D. S. Massey, "Determinants of English Proficiency among Mexican Migrants to the United States," *International Migration Review* 31, no. 1 (Spring 1997): 28–50.

10. J. S. Reichman, "Language-Specific Response Patterns and Subjective Assessment of Health: A Sociolinguistic Analysis," *Hispanic Journal of Behavioral Sciences* 19, no. 3 (August 1997): 358.

11. According to a 1999 study by Orfield and Yun, Latino/a segregation in public schools continues to occur where there is a large Latino/a or Spanish-speaking population, and this experience is similar to that of African Americans. See G. Orfield and J. T. Yun, "Resegregation in American Schools," The Civil Rights Project, Harvard University, http://www.law.harvard.edu/.

12. M. Barrera, *Race and Class in the Southwest: A Theory of Racial Inequality* (Notre Dame, IN: University of Notre Dame Press, 1979), 76–89.

13. L. Pulido, *Environmentalism and Economic Justice: Two Chicano Struggles in the Southwest* (Tucson: University of Arizona Press, 1996).

Suggested Readings

Estrada, A. L. "Mexican Americans and Historical Trauma Theory: A Theoretical Perspective." *Journal of Ethnicity in Substance Abuse* 8, no. 3 (2009): 330–40.

González, G. G. *Chicano Education in the Era of Segregation*. Philadelphia: Balch Institute Press, 1990.

Griswold del Castillo, R. *North to Aztlán: A History of Mexican Americans in the United States*. New York: Twayne Publishers, 1996.

———. *The Treaty of Guadalupe Hidalgo: A Legacy of Conflict*. Norman: University of Oklahoma Press, 1990.

Gutiérrez, D. G. *Walls and Mirrors*. Berkeley: University of California Press, 1995.

Hamamoto, D., and R. Torres. *New American Destinies: A Reader in Contemporary Asian and Latino Immigration*. New York: Routledge, 1997.

Hispanic Americas: A Statistical Sourcebook. Boulder, CO: Numbers and Concepts, 1991.

Martínez, O. J. *Border People: Life and Society in the U.S.-Mexico Borderlands*. Tucson: University of Arizona Press, 1994.

Pulido, L. *Environmentalism and Economic Justice: Two Chicano Struggles in the Southwest*. Tucson: University of Arizona Press, 1996.

Romero, M., P. Hodagneu-Sotelo, and V. Ortiz. *Challenging Fronteras*. New York: Routledge, 1997.

San Miguel, G. *"Let All of Them Take Heed": Mexican Americans and the Campaign for Educational Equality in Texas, 1910–1981*. Austin: University of Texas Press, 1987.

Tienda, M., and L. Jensen. "Immigration and Social Program Participation: Dispelling the Myth of Dependency." *Social Science Research* 15 (1986): 372–400.

U.S. Department of Commerce, Economics, and Statistics Administration, Bureau of the Census. *We the American Hispanics*. Washington, DC: Government Printing Office, 1993.

Vélez Ibáñez, C. G. *Border Visions: Mexican Cultures of the Southwest United States*. Tucson: University of Arizona Press, 1996.

Chapter 2

The Health Status of Mexican Americans

"It's about Having a Healthy Body"

Latinos now make up the largest ethnic minority group in the United States, particularly in the Southwest. Yet it is very troubling to find that there is still relatively little information on the health status of the overall group or the four major Latino subgroups (Mexican Americans, Central and South Americans, Puerto Ricans, and Cubans). One may well ask how the U.S. government or individual states can make informed health policy decisions regarding Latinos when there is such a paucity of knowledge. In this chapter, we highlight what is known about the health status of Mexican Americans and discuss changes that need to be made in order to meet the health-care needs of this large group.

The Historical Context of Health and Disease

To understand contemporary Mexican American concepts of disease and healing, we must first examine the historical context of several core indigenous (native) beliefs and their **syncretism**, or merging, with those of the colonial Spanish. The Indians of Mesoamerica,[1] influenced primarily by the Mixteca or Aztecs, believed in three animistic forces (multiple souls) that have relevance in contemporary Mexican folk medicine.[2] According to Ortiz de Montellano (1990), in Mesoamerican culture, a person's health depended on the relative amounts of each soul at a given time and on the maintenance of balance among them. *Tonalli*, believed to be located in the head, provided a vital hot force. It imparted bravery, vigor, and warmth and made growth possible. Involuntary loss of one's Tonalli could cause illness or even death. *Teyolia*, believed to be located in the heart, provided vitality, knowledge, and vocational ability. The Aztecs believed the heart to be the center of thought and personality. This soul, unlike Tonalli, could be separated from the body only at the time of death and was known as the soul "that goes beyond after death." The third animistic force was *Ihiyotl*. Thought to be located in the liver, Ihiyotl provided vigor, passions, and feelings such as desire, envy, and anger. Sins, particularly of a sexual nature, were believed to harm the liver and make it emit Ihiyotl, which could harm others. The Aztecs believed health to be holistic. To stay healthy one had to be in equilibrium, do things in moderation, and perform one's duty. States of illness and health were closely related to a condition of equilibrium or disequilibrium. Health required a person to maintain equilibrium physically, in social relations, and with the deities. Causes of disease included supernatural (religious), magical, and natural (physical) sources, but all were intertwined. The Aztecs had their own system of "hot" and "cold" diseases, similar to but different in important ways from the Spanish model.

The Spanish brought with them to the Americas concepts of disease and healing based on **Hippocratic-Galenic beliefs,** and to some extent, concepts derived from Arabic medicine. A major part of this belief system was the existence of four humors, or liquids, in the body—black bile, yellow bile, phlegm, and blood. The relative levels of the humors in a person's body determined his or her temperament and physical and mental characteristics and had the potential to cause disease. Additionally, given the pervasive belief in witches and witchcraft during the sixteenth century, the Spanish also believed in the supernatural causation of disease through hexes and spells. The most important concepts derived from the Spanish were the concepts of "hot" and "cold" diseases derived from Hippocratic-Galenic medicine. Vasodilation (opening of the blood vessels) and a high metabolic rate characterized "hot" diseases, whereas vasoconstriction (narrowing of the blood vessels) and a low metabolic rate characterized "cold" diseases. Examples of "hot" conditions include pregnancy, hypertension, diabetes, acid indigestion, **susto, mal de ojo,** and **bilis.** Examples of "cold" conditions include menstrual cramps, pneumonia, colic, **empacho,** and **frío de la matriz.** "Cold" remedies usually treat "hot" diseases and "hot" remedies usually treat "cold" diseases.

It is important to keep this historical perspective in mind when examining the health status of Mexican Americans. In particular, contemporary concepts of illness and wellness are closely linked to several aspects of historical beliefs, especially in terms of the common folk illnesses found among Mexican Americans.

The Sociocultural Basis of Health and Disease

> I do have to say that I believe that it [language] definitely had to have been
> an issue when I was growing up because we did live in poverty, but my
> grandparents were never on welfare or any kind of assistance. . . . [N]ow
> that I think back, they didn't consider looking into those options. I'm sure
> that we would have definitely qualified because we had a house full of chil-
> dren. (María L., 44)

Health does not exist in isolation from socioeconomic or cultural factors.
In fact, socioeconomic status profoundly influences health status, both
positively and negatively. Cultural values, beliefs, and attitudes influence
help-seeking behaviors. There is no question that income, educational
attainment, and poverty levels are closely linked to health. Mexican Americans as a group have lower incomes, lower educational attainment, and
higher poverty rates than non-Latino whites. But how exactly do these
socioeconomic differences affect health status?

Several socioeconomic characteristics of the Mexican-origin population have a harmful effect on both its general health-care behaviors and
its general health status. Low income, substandard housing, inadequate
or unsanitary living facilities, lack of formal education, ethnic segregation and discrimination, poor nutrition, and stress can and do affect the
health of Mexican Americans in a number of ways. Overcrowded housing
and lack of appropriate sanitation increase exposure to infectious diseases.
Low education levels result in decreased awareness of health promotion
and disease prevention activities (such as diet, exercise, and reducing one's
risk of exposure to diseases). Additionally, these barriers limit utilization
of health care and prescription medications and contribute to institutionalized racism and discrimination. Finally, they increase the probability that
an individual will choose alternative forms of health care that may be inef-
fective or even harmful. Many diseases found among the Mexican-origin
population are associated with poverty. Bacterial and parasitic diseases and
tuberculosis, for example, are related to overcrowding, poor nutrition, and
inadequate housing and sanitation.

> When I found out that my uterus had fallen and tipped, I was told by
> someone that maybe I could get massaged and that they could lift it up. . . .
> Everybody wants to try to avoid any type of surgery at all costs and if there
> is another alternative that you have heard about then you kind of want

to give it a try. . . . I had gone to a *santero* [spiritual healer], I was taking a friend, and while he was there [I] decided to go ahead. I asked him if he felt it was a good idea to have the surgery and he said it wasn't and he is the one that suggested for me to seek someone that could massage and put it back. (María L., 44)

Cultural influences also affect Mexican American health and health-care behavior. Cultural values such as machismo among men and marianismo among women influence decisions to seek health care, symptom recognition, and disease management. Cultural values such as familismo, **personalismo**, confianza, **dignidad**, and respeto affect the provider-patient relationship and help determine whether a patient stays in treatment or follows prescribed regimens. Cultural beliefs regarding health and illness shape how a person communicates individual health problems, perceives and interprets symptoms, chooses when and where to go for care, decides how long to stay in care, and evaluates the care received.

Perhaps the most widely examined cultural concept in relation to the health status of Mexican Americans is acculturation. Acculturation is a dynamic process. It signifies dual learning and the blending of mainstream (European American) cultural values, beliefs, attitudes, and behaviors with those originating in Mexican culture. Acculturation is often measured by indicators such as language preference and use (Spanish or English), ethnic identification (Mexican, Mexican American, Chicano/a, or Mexicano/a), birthplace (Mexico or the United States), and generational status (first, second, or higher order).[3] Acculturation is believed to influence behaviors, attitudes and beliefs, and values held by members of the Mexican-origin population. Using this concept, health researchers have found that less acculturated Mexican-origin individuals tend to have inaccurate health information and lack relevant health knowledge regarding symptom recognition. At the same time, research has also shown that more acculturated Mexican Americans tend to have poorer nutrition and engage in more health-related risk behaviors such as use of tobacco, alcohol, and drugs. However, a major problem with this concept is that greater acculturation is often associated with higher educational and income levels (both of which are known to influence general health status), as well as access to and use of health-care services. Therefore, given that persons of lower socioeconomic status are also more likely to be less acculturated (and vice versa) it is necessary to disentangle the effects of socioeconomic status and acculturation level.

Health Promotion and Disease Prevention in the Mexican American Community

> At eighteen years old . . . doctors detected my illness and noticed that my illness was spreading and not stopping. The illness had reached my kidneys. I had weighed one hundred pounds, and my kidneys stopped functioning. I went through very hard times due to the symptoms of my illness. I was not able to do anything on my own, and my family helped me. . . . It was very hard, we spent about ten years paying medical bills. (Lorena B., 48)

The development and implementation of health promotion and disease prevention programs in Mexican-origin communities are critical. However, to develop such programs we need a thorough understanding of the **epidemiological** (distributional) factors that contribute to disease, the cultural factors that weaken or enhance disease prevention, and the socioeconomic profile of the community to be targeted.

Researchers have suggested several acculturation models to explain variations in disease **incidence** and **prevalence**. These two most common measures of disease rates, incidence and prevalence, refer, respectively, to the number of new cases of a disease and the total number of cases of a disease. The majority of these models relate health outcomes to **acculturative stress**, the stress of adapting one's culture to the mainstream culture.[4] The simple acculturation model proposes that acculturation is not in itself stressful and therefore is not associated with increased incidence or prevalence of disease. The acculturative stress models suggest two opposite outcomes: either less acculturated Latinos, because of their health values and health behaviors, will show higher incidence and prevalence of disease than more acculturated Latinos; or alternatively, more acculturated Latinos, due to cultural loss, will show higher incidence and prevalence of disease than less acculturated Latinos. The bicultural model suggests that Latinos who retain traditional cultural values and behaviors while also being able to interact with the dominant culture will have better health status than both poorly and highly acculturated Latinos.

In spelling out causal factors, it is important to understand key epidemiological concepts such as incidence, prevalence, **relative risk**, and **attributable risk**. Very generally, relative risk measures the likelihood that members in a group will contract a disease, and attributable risk measures the number of illnesses caused by exposure to a disease. It is also critical to know which risk factors contribute to specific diseases and what the prevalence of these risk factors are in the Mexican-origin community. For example, cardiovascular disease (heart disease and heart attack) is the leading cause of mortality (death) among Mexican American adults. Several important **modifiable risk factors** contribute to the incidence of cardiovascular disease, such as high cholesterol levels, smoking, lack of exercise, and obesity. Research shows that these risk factors are more prevalent among Mexican Americans than among non-Latino whites. This information helps us target the behaviors that contribute to these risk factors.

Cultural factors that weaken or enhance disease prevention efforts include gender role concepts such as machismo and marianismo, cultural beliefs regarding effective cures and treatments, and cultural values or attitudes about the body and the disease itself. For example, breast cancer is one of the most commonly diagnosed cancers among Mexican American women. Yet the cultural value of marianismo dictates that a woman should place the health-care needs of other family members before her own. Fear and anxiety about cancer may act as another barrier to early screening. Cultural values related to avoidance of touching the body or allowing someone else to view or touch the body (even a health professional) may prevent some Mexican-origin women from performing breast self-exams, agreeing to clinical breast exams, or obtaining a mammography.

One of the most widely used public health models of disease prevention includes the concepts of **primary, secondary,** and **tertiary prevention**. Each of these levels of prevention is directly linked to the **natural history of disease**. The natural history of disease has four stages: susceptibility (e.g., risk factors), presymptomatic disease (e.g., early signs of disease), clinical disease (e.g., recognizable signs and symptoms of disease), and disability (e.g., reduced function or impairment). Primary prevention focuses on addressing modifiable risk factors in the susceptibility stage to prevent the disease from progressing. The ultimate goal of primary prevention is to reduce the incidence (the number of new cases) of a disease. Secondary prevention targets individuals who are beginning to show presymptomatic or symptomatic signs of disease. They receive services such as early detection and risk-reduction education designed to slow or stop the progression of the disease. The goal of secondary prevention is to reduce the prevalence of disease (the total number of people affected by a disease). Lastly, tertiary prevention focuses on those individuals who have the disease in its full clinical stage, resulting in some disability. The goal of tertiary prevention is to restore health and reduce the level of disability caused by the disease.

Socioeconomic factors are important because they contribute to the incidence and prevalence of disease, as well as providing us with information on which subgroups to target and in what form intervention should be delivered. For example, imagine that a community assessment finds that the majority of Mexican-origin people living in a particular area are monolingual Spanish speakers and have low literacy rates in both Spanish and English. These factors mean that one must present the risk-reduction message in Spanish and through media outlets that do not depend solely on reading ability.

Understanding epidemiological factors, cultural factors, and socioeconomic factors is just the beginning. These factors must now be used to develop culturally competent health promotion and disease prevention programs targeting Mexican Americans. (For a thorough discussion of **cultural competency**, see chapter 5.) Here we will briefly highlight important elements needed for the development of culturally competent interventions that focus on risk reduction.

The placement of the program for health promotion and disease prevention is critical. It must be in a geographic setting that is accessible and acceptable to Mexican Americans. The program must be community-based, that is, set within the Mexican-origin community. Care must be taken to ensure that the **subjective culture** (attitudes, values, beliefs, etc.) of Mexican Americans is well represented.[5] The program must be staffed with bicultural and bilingual individuals. Client-staff interactions must be guided by core Mexican and Mexican American cultural values such as **simpatía**, personalismo, dignidad, respeto, and confianza. Depending on the specific disease and modifiable risk factors targeted, concepts such as familismo, religiosity, and spirituality may play important roles as well.

An essential component of any prevention program is community empowerment, or strengthening the community's ability to meet its own needs. One model that encompasses this underlying goal is the Nuestro Bienestar model developed by the Center for Health Policy Development in San Antonio, Texas. This model is guided by **razalogía**, a community development approach originating in the 1970s.[6] According to Andrade and Doria-Ortiz, "The *razalogía* model takes as its mission the empowerment of *raza* communities, and it challenges each individual community member to identify, contrast and compare, and then reject concepts and behaviors which weaken their resolution to act on behalf of the community's *bienestar* (health, well-being, strength, unity)."[7] Other aspects of community empowerment include having an advisory board composed of community members and obtaining a consensus from the community on the importance of targeting specific risk factors or diseases. A useful guide to follow when developing an intervention is Freire's problem-posing method. This method involves having community members identify the problem, analyze its causes, and develop solutions.[8]

The Health Status of Mexican American Sociodemographic Subgroups

> We did live in a poor area, and when my dad left we became poorer. My dad left when I was seven, so after seven years old when the electricity went out, we used candles. When there was no food, we didn't eat. When the window broke, it stayed broke. When our car broke down, it stayed in the parking lot. Things just stayed bad and they didn't get better. . . . It was really hard for me to believe that anything was ever going to change in my life. I used to wonder when my dad was going to come home, wonder when days would change and when life was ever going to get better. It got a lot worse before it ever got better. (Danny F., 36)

Children and Youth

In the United States, health and demographic data is collected between birth and seventeen years of age. This age group is often referred to as the child population. However, youth data partially intersects this age group. The term "youth" refers to the period between childhood and adulthood. It typically encompasses the ages between sixteen and twenty-four.[9]

The health of Mexican American children and youth is inextricably linked to the socioeconomic and cultural factors affecting their parents and families. A useful heuristic (problem-solving) approach is to examine the socio-economic, institutional, and cultural contexts that influence the health of children and youth, acknowledging that all three contexts are interrelated.[10]

The socioeconomic context includes factors such as poverty status, educational attainment, and median household income. As noted in chapter 1, a significant number of Mexican-origin families live below the **federal poverty level**. In 2009, more than one-fourth of all Latinos were living in poverty, which was more than twice the rate of non-Latino whites. Further, almost one-third of Latino children (those under eighteen years of age) were living in poverty. This proportion increases when only female-headed households are considered, showing that approximately 39 percent of Latino children in this situation were living in poverty in 2009.[11] The fact that higher rates of poverty are found among female-headed households than in other household types is referred to as the "**feminization of poverty.**" The educational attainment of parents is another important factor that may harm or aid the health of children and youth. Among Latinos twenty-five years of age or older, 39 percent have less than twelve years of education, and it is well established that income increases with educational attainment. Results from the 2011 American Community Survey Report show that synthetic work-life earnings (i.e., the expected earnings over a forty-year period for the population between the ages of twenty-five and sixty-four based on annual earnings from a single (cross-sectional) point in time) for Latinos increases threefold with number of years of education.[12]

The institutional context of health involves many of the factors identified in the next chapter concerning health-care access and includes the ability to obtain and pay for health care and the availability of linguistically and culturally competent health-care providers. Some of the more specific factors include health insurance coverage, having a regular source of care or a particular provider, and barriers to health-care use.

The Commonwealth Fund 2001 Health Care Quality Survey found that only 56 percent of Latinos reported being satisfied by the care they had received in the past two years; 40 percent of Latinos felt that they could get proper medical care when necessary; 14 percent of Latinos reported depending on the emergency room for care or didn't have a source for care at all; and only 57 percent of Latinos reported having a regular doctor.

Clearly, parents of Mexican American children are at a distinct disadvantage relative to non-Latino whites in reference to the institutional context of health care. Factors such as state and federal policies that limit access to health care for undocumented Mexican immigrants but also serve to institutionalize discriminatory practices by health-care facilities are also a problem. These discriminatory practices present barriers to legal immigrants and native-born Mexican Americans as well as undocumented immigrants.

The cultural context of health among Mexican American children and youth involves familial cultural practices and values that either promote health or detract from it. Mexican-origin families often have hierarchical family roles, extended family systems, and gender role expectations.

Mexican-origin children usually acculturate or adapt to the U.S. mainstream society more quickly and easily than their parents do. Consequently, there may be more intergenerational conflict between parents and children in terms of appropriate gender and age-specific roles. Additionally, because many Mexican American families have more than one child in the home, an older child may be expected to care for younger ones and to assist parents in their acculturation to mainstream society. This can result in the so-called parentification of children. That is, too much responsibility is placed on youth without additional familial support or guidance. The effects of these stressors can lead to mental health and substance-abuse problems as children mature.

EMERGENT HEALTH ISSUES FOR MEXICAN AMERICAN CHILDREN

Several important health issues affecting Mexican-origin children are highlighted in this chapter; they are underimmunization, obesity, and oral health.

> The issue of transportation was a big issue. My mother depended upon social service agencies, charitable hospitals . . . she depended on the sisters of charity to obtain health care for all of us. For immunizations we had to go to the clinics. . . . We would walk to the clinic. We would have to traverse railroad tracks, busy intersections, and she had all these kids, and we just had to stick together as much as possible. My mother was very determined; even though it was difficult to access, she never failed to . . . get us necessary immunizations and so forth. (Gracie S., 46)

The underimmunization of Mexican American children is an important health issue. Lack of needed immunizations may prevent them from being enrolled in school, but more importantly it contributes to increased communicable disease incidence, prevalence, and morbidity (rate of illness). Most childhood communicable diseases are preventable with appropriate immunization. In 2009, only about 74 percent of Latino children between nineteen and thirty-five months of age had been vaccinated for the combined series of diphtheria-tetanus-pertussis (DTP) vaccine, polio vaccine, measles-containing vaccine, Haemophilus influenza type b (Hib) vaccine, and the hepatitis B vaccine. Latino children living in poverty had significantly lower vaccination rates than those living at or above the poverty level: 74 percent versus 80 percent, respectively.[13] Underimmunization is an even greater problem in the U.S.-Mexico border area.[14] The low level of childhood immunization among Mexican Americans reflects a number of underlying issues: lack of knowledge regarding immunization efficacy, lack of health-care access, and lack of affordable health care.

Obesity (being significantly overweight) is another important indicator of the future health status of Mexican-origin children and youth. Obesity is a primary modifiable risk factor for the development of diabetes, heart disease, cerebrovascular disease (stroke and high blood pressure), and cancer. Available data indicate that Mexican American children are significantly more overweight than non-Latino white children. For example, 26.8 percent of Mexican American boys between the ages of twelve and nineteen were obese, compared to 16.7 percent of non-Latino white boys of the same age. Moreover, 17.4 percent of Mexican American girls between the ages of twelve and nineteen were obese compared to 14.5 percent of non-Latina white girls of the same age range. In Mexican American infants to children two years of age, 15.7 percent of either gender had high weight-to-height ratios.[15] Obesity and above-average weight are risk factors that can be decreased through increased exercise, better nutrition, and environmental changes that support access to healthy foods and healthy eating behaviors.

An exemplary program that aims to understand and aid Mexican American children with overweight and obesity risk factors is the Niños Sanos, Familia Sana program supported by the United States Department of Agriculture's National Institute of Food and Agriculture, or USDA-NIFA, and implemented through a research team at UC Davis. This program works with Mexican American children (ages 3–8) in California's rural Central Valley to intervene in and help correct and prevent obesity. Intervention programs include education on eating right, exercise, economic incentives, and community-based initiatives to help support families in making the right food and exercise choices for healthy living. These family choices are supported and sustained by creating a healthier environment for these families. Important elements of the program include creating culturally appropriate education programs for communities and increasing the number of culturally competent students (undergraduate, graduate, and professional) that can understand the issues of this community in order to better serve them. Niños Sanos, Familia Sana utilizes community input and participation to both understand community needs and give the community a sense of ownership over the program and intervention methods.

Oral health is another important issue affecting Mexican-origin children. In general, Latinos have higher rates of periodontal (gum) disease than do non-Latino whites. Periodontal disease such as gingivitis (redness and swelling of the gums) is prevalent among Mexican American children. The Burden of Oral Disease tool from the Centers for Disease Control and Prevention (CDC) shows that 69 percent of Mexican American children between the ages of six and eight experience tooth decay, and 42 percent are untreated. A report by the National Center for Health Statistics (NCHS) (2007) indicated that approximately half of all Mexican American children between the ages of two and eleven have decayed or filled surfaces in their primary teeth.[16] These findings point to future trends of tooth decay, tooth loss, and severe periodontal disease among Mexican Americans as they age.

MEXICAN AMERICAN ADOLESCENTS

> I would say that the use of drugs and alcohol . . . has bothered me ever since I was going to school. I could possibly have respiratory problems because I have smoked quite a lot . . . marijuana was what I smoked the most. (Enrique A., 30)

> My mother . . . left to go take care of her mom when I was fourteen. . . . I never wanted to be in a gang and I never wanted to use drugs or alcohol. . . . There was substance abuse in my house. There was violence and it became a hopeless place, and a lot of my friends started using and I never wanted to use. (Danny F., 36)

Mexican-origin adolescents engage in a number of risk behaviors that may be detrimental to their present and future health status as well as their future socioeconomic status. Again, the social, cultural, and institutional context of health makes an important contribution to understanding the health status of Mexican American adolescents. One can readily see that the same issues that influence children's health also affect the health of adolescents.

Diabetes is a metabolic disorder that results from the body's inability either to convert glucose into energy due to lack of insulin (Type I diabetes) or to adequately use the insulin produced (Type II diabetes). As a consequence, glucose builds up in the blood, which can lead to a diabetic coma. The prevalence of Type II diabetes (**non-insulin-dependent diabetes mellitus** or NIDDM), which is often triggered by lifestyle factors such as poor diet and obesity, is increasing among Mexican Americans. Part of this increase is due to the early onset of NIDDM among Mexican American adolescents.[17] Neufeld and colleagues found that 45 percent of the incident cases (new cases) of NIDDM in one provider setting were among youth. Modifiable risk factors for diabetes include obesity and being overweight, high dietary fat and low fiber intake, and a sedentary lifestyle.[18] All of these factors are reportedly higher in Mexican American adolescents than in non-Latino white adolescents.

Early sexual activity and teen pregnancy are other important issues that Mexican American adolescents face. Adolescence is a time of rapid physiological maturation. Mexican American girls reach puberty sooner than do non-Latino white girls. This earlier age of menarche, when females begin their menstrual period, is a factor in both the higher fertility rate found among Mexican Americans and the higher teen-pregnancy rate. Available research suggests that even though Mexican American girls have a lower reported rate of sexual activity in comparison to non-Latino white girls, they tend to use contraceptives less.[19] This puts them at greater risk for pregnancy, which may affect continued growth and development. It also places them at risk for sexually transmitted diseases (STDs) such as HIV/AIDS, human papillomavirus (HPV), syphilis, gonorrhea, trichomonas, and chlamydia. Lack of contraceptive use by both adolescent Mexican American boys and girls can certainly lead to unintended pregnancies and a life of low socioeconomic status resulting from dropping out of school or not being able to find well-paying jobs.

Motor vehicle accidents, homicides, and suicides are leading causes of death among all adolescents, including Mexican-origin teens. While the mortality rates for motor vehicle accidents are similar to those of non-Latino whites, Mexican American adolescents have a higher prevalence of homicides and suicides. The homicide rate among Latino males between the ages of fourteen and nineteen is over seven times higher than that of non-Latino whites in that age group.[20] High school Latina female adolescents are about 40 percent more likely to report having attempted suicide than their non-Latino white counterparts.[21]

Mexican American Adults

As Mexican Americans move from adolescence into adulthood a number of changes in cellular structures of the body and organs take place. Most of these changes are directly attributable to lifestyle behaviors during adolescence. This section will briefly highlight key morbidity and mortality characteristics of adults.

Morbidity and Mortality

> If a person doesn't have health insurance, they don't have access to a provider. . . . Unless they really know what's really going [on] with the community . . . if they don't have proper insurance they're not going for their preventative health exams so that'll hinder someone [who] is developing some type of disease. It is not going to be caught on time. They'll probably be diagnosed with later stages of the disease like my mother. . . . She was diagnosed with breast cancer at her later stages, it wasn't at a point where it could be caught [i.e., arrested]. So if a person doesn't have health insurance and they're not going for their routine health physicals then a person will become sicker. (María P., 31)

The general health status of Mexican American adults is correlated with educational and income levels. For example, among Mexican Americans between the ages of forty-five and sixty-four with fewer than twelve years of education, 30 percent rated their health as fair or poor compared to only 15 percent of those with twelve or more years of education.

Chronic diseases are directly related to illness, hospitalization, and limitation of activity. Among Mexican-origin adults, major chronic diseases include metabolic syndrome, NIDDM, heart disease, stroke, cancer, and HIV disease.

Metabolic syndrome represents a cluster of risk factors that are directly linked to NIDDM. The major characteristics of metabolic syndrome include insulin resistance, abdominal obesity, elevated blood pressure, and lipid abnormalities such as elevated levels of triglycerides, and low levels of high-density lipoprotein (HDL) cholesterol. Approximately one in three Latino men and women over twenty years of age have metabolic syndrome.

NIDDM is one of the more prevalent diseases found among Mexican Americans; it was the fifth leading cause of death among Latinos in 2011. However, the nature of NIDDM means that it is often a contributing factor in deaths due to heart disease and kidney failure.

> The most important factor is to have early detection for your health. . . .
> [A]fter I was pronounced with diabetes I wasn't having a yearly checkup

and worrying about how do I feel. I learned through my experience with my illness that you have to have a yearly checkup. . . . [N]ow my main goal is not to go on insulin. So it depends on my diet, on my medication, and my monthly blood test. (Yolanda N., 52)

It is estimated that more than one in every ten Mexican Americans over twenty years of age has diabetes.[22] Diabetes data and trends from CDC show that the prevalence of diagnosed diabetes is 9.1 percent for Mexican Americans compared to 5.3 percent for non-Latino whites. The prevalence of diabetes also increases with age. The prevalence of diabetes was 35.5 percent for Mexican Americans between the ages of sixty-five and seventy-four.

Evidence from the CDC Behavioral Risk Factor Survey suggests that both the prevalence of NIDDM and risk factors for its development are high for southwestern Latinos compared to non-Latino whites.[23] The prevalence of obesity among Latinos residing in the five southwestern states of Arizona, California, Colorado, New Mexico, and Texas ranged from a low of 25.1 percent (Colorado) to a high of 32.3 percent (Texas). The prevalence of NIDDM in the five southwestern states ranged from a low of 5.9 percent (Colorado) to a high of 10.4 percent (Texas).

Risk factors for diabetes include obesity and being overweight, metabolic syndrome, impaired glucose tolerance, insulin resistance, and a family history of diabetes. The prevalence of obesity is higher among Mexican Americans than among non-Latino whites, which contributes to the higher incidence of diabetes.[24] Also, overweight Mexican-origin women have a higher risk of developing diabetes during pregnancy (gestational diabetes) than do overweight non-Latino white women. The prevalence of diabetes among Mexican Americans whose parents have diabetes is twice that of Mexican Americans with no family history of diabetes. Impaired glucose tolerance is higher among Mexican Americans than among non-Latino whites. The CDC's publication "National Diabetes Fact Sheet, 2011" reported a prevalence rate of 13.3 percent among Mexican Americans compared to 7.1 percent among non-Latino whites aged twenty and older (after adjusting for population age differences).[25] Two population-based studies have demonstrated higher insulin levels among Mexican Americans than among non-Latino whites.[26] These higher insulin levels may reflect resistance to insulin reception in tissues due to increased adiposity (fat content) and are predictive of NIDDM incidence.

Complications resulting from late diagnosis and poor medical management of NIDDM are also more prevalent in Mexican Americans than in non-Latino whites. The prevalence of proteinuria, a key indicator of kidney damage, is more common among Mexican Americans, and the rate of diabetic retinopathy, an eye disease often leading to blindness, is more than twice that of non-Latino whites. Additionally, Mexican Americans with NIDDM have a higher rate of peripheral vascular disease (damage to the blood vessels), leading to amputation of the feet or legs, than is found in non-Hispanic whites. Taken together, the increasing incidence and prevalence of NIDDM will lead to premature death among Mexican Americans if it is not detected early and appropriately managed. The key to reducing the incidence of NIDDM among Mexican Americans is to target modifiable risk factors—obesity and being overweight—through increased exercise and better-quality diets. Persons with a known familial history of diabetes should obtain appropriate screening for diabetes. By reducing the incidence of NIDDM, we can also reduce its prevalence and health consequences.

Cardiovascular disease (CVD) includes heart disease, congestive heart failure, and myocardial infarction (heart attack). Heart disease is the leading cause of death among all racial/ethnic groups in the United States. Cerebrovascular disease includes hypertension (high blood pressure) and stroke and is the fourth leading cause of death among Latinos. Major contributing factors to the incidence of cardiovascular and cerebrovascular diseases include atherosclerosis (hardening of the arteries), obesity, being overweight, high cholesterol, poor diet, lack of exercise, cigarette smoking, family history, and NIDDM.

Atherosclerosis is the underlying condition for both cardiovascular and cerebrovascular disease. It occurs when the inner layers of the artery walls become thickened by a buildup of fatty deposits and other substances. As the inner wall of the artery thickens, there is less space for the blood to flow through, resulting in a diminished blood supply. Symptoms of reduced blood flow include chest pain and hypertension. A stroke results when an artery in the brain is either ruptured or clogged by a blood clot (thrombus), a wandering clot (embolus), or atherosclerosis plaque. Cells in the affected region of the brain die within minutes, resulting in disability. Bleeding in the brain caused by an aneurysm (weakening and ballooning of a blood vessel) is the other principal cause of stroke. This type of stroke is the result of a ruptured blood vessel that bleeds into the brain tissue (called cerebral hemorrhage).

Research has shown that Mexican Americans have similar prevalence rates to non-Latino whites of elevated cholesterol and slightly higher rates of hypertension. For example, the 2012 Morbidity and Mortality Chart Book found the prevalence of elevated cholesterol to be about 17 percent and 14 percent among Mexican American men and women, respectively, compared to about 14 percent and 17 percent among non-Latino white men and women.[27] The rate of hypertension was about 21.8 percent and 20.7 percent among Mexican American men and women, respectively, compared to about 27.4 percent and 23.1 percent among non-Latino white men and women. Findings from the National Health and Nutrition Examination Survey (NHANES, 2003–2006) show that compared to non-Latino whites and African Americans, Mexican Americans have lower rates of hypertension awareness, treatment, and control, which can lead to increases in the incidence of, the prevalence of, and mortality from hypertension-related diseases.[28]

Nevertheless, deaths due to CVD are lower for Latinos than for non-Latino whites and African Americans. In 2006, the mortality rate for CVD was 27 per 100,000 for Latino men, compared with 33.3 per 100,000 for non-Latino white males and 32.3 percent for African American males. Latina women also had lower CVD death rates than non-Latina white and African American women.[29]

> As we all know, stress is the causing factor for many diseases. . . . I developed pretty large fibroids in my uterus and as a result I had to have a hysterectomy because I was losing a lot of hemoglobin and I became acutely anemic in the process, to the point where I had to have a transfusion because of it. (Carmen G., 49)

Cancer is the second leading cause of death among Latinos. The three most common types of cancers found in Mexican-origin men are lung cancer, cancer of the prostate, and colon cancer.[30] The three most common types of cancer found in Mexican-origin women are breast cancer, lung cancer, and colorectal cancer. The incidence rates of lung cancer among men and women is approximately 47.6 and 25.2 per 100,000, respectively, which are about 45 percent lower than the rates for non-Latino white men and women. The five-year survival rates for lung cancer are about 9 percent for Mexican American men and 15 percent for Mexican American women, which are similar to the rates for non-Latino whites. The major risk factor for lung cancer is cigarette smoking, which accounts for 87 percent of the attributable risk.

The colorectal cancer incidence rates for Latino men and women are 50 and 35.1 per 100,000, respectively, which again are lower than the rates for non-Latino whites and African Americans. Colorectal cancer incidence rates are about 20 percent lower among Latinos than among non-Latino whites. However, five-year survival rates are slightly lower for Mexican American males than for non-Latino white males (41 percent compared to 46 percent) and are similar for Mexican American and non-Latino white females (50 percent). The major risk factors for colorectal cancer are a low-fiber, high-fat diet; low intake of fruits and vegetables; physical inactivity; a family history of colorectal cancer; or a history of polyps and inflammatory bowel disease.

Among Latino men, prostate cancer has an incidence rate of 131.1 per 100,000, which is slightly lower than the rates for non-Latino white males (141 per 100,000) and African American males (228.7 per 100,000). Mortality rates in 2010 for prostate cancer are also slightly lower for Mexican Americans than for non-Latino whites, at approximately 18.0 per 100,000 and 20.1 per 100,000, respectively. Causes of prostate cancer are largely unknown, but some research suggests that occupational exposure, a diet high in fat, early sexual activity, an increase in sex hormones, and a family history contribute to the incidence of prostate cancer.

> There were complications due to the loss of blood that I had prior to surgery and during surgery and then when I first was able to get in, the doctor requested was not the doctor I saw. . . . I got a referral to see a gynecologist and again with him I waited for about an hour and saw him for five minutes and I was really concerned because I didn't feel that he took time to get to know my case and who I was. (Carmen G., 49)

Aside from colorectal cancer, the two most prevalent cancers found among Mexican-origin women are breast cancer and lung cancer. Latina women have a significantly lower incidence rate of breast cancer than do non-Latina white women, at 90.2 per 100,000 and 123.5 per 100,000, respectively. However, the 2010 mortality rates were only slightly lower for Mexican American women in comparison to non-Latina white women, at 14.4 per 100,000 and 21.9 per 100,000, respectively. The major risk factors for breast cancer include first-term pregnancy after age thirty, obesity after menopause, alcohol consumption, high-fat diet, lack of physical activity, and family history. The major risk factor for lung cancer is the same as that for men, as described on the previous page.

Overall cancer incidence is lower for Latinos than for non-Latino whites and African Americans. However, Latinos have higher incidence rates of liver, stomach, and gallbladder cancers than do non-Latino whites. More research is needed to determine causal factors related to these types of cancers, such as the association between a type of bacteria known as *Helicobacter pylori* (*H. pylori*) and stomach cancer.

One of the chief methods for lowering the incidence and prevalence of all the common cancers found among Mexican Americans is early detection through appropriate screening. Although this appears to be an easy solution, numerous sociocultural factors interfere with its achievement. These include a general lack of knowledge about recognizing symptoms and effective treatments, a lack of access to health care and use of preventative health services, and attitudes and values regarding the human body, especially those areas most affected by these cancers—the breast, cervix, and prostate.

Studies by Johnson-Kozlow and colleagues, using the 2005 California Health Interview Survey, found that 43 percent of Mexican Americans were likely to not have had any colorectal screening, compared to 22 percent of non-Latino whites.[31] Clearly, to reduce the incidence and prevalence of these major forms of cancer among Mexican Americans, knowledge of cancer screenings must increase.

The CDC reports that of the 197,090 diagnoses of HIV infection between 2008 and 2011, Latinos accounted for 21 percent.[32] Sixteen percent of those diagnosed were women, and 18 percent were attributed to heterosexual contact. Among Latinos, the mode by which HIV, which causes AIDS, is transmitted varies by place of birth.

For example, in 2011 among Mexican-born males, 81.9 percent who contracted the virus were men who have sex with men (MSMs), 4.7 percent were injection drug users (IDUs), and 3 percent were MSMs and IDUs; 10.4 percent contracted the virus through heterosexual contact. In contrast Puerto Rican–born males acquired the virus primarily through MSM (50.1 percent), heterosexual contact (23.5 percent), and injection drug use (22.9 percent). We see similar results for Puerto Rican women, who acquired the virus primarily through sex with an HIV-positive male (82.6 percent) and injection drug use (17.2 percent). Among non-Latino white women, 75 percent acquired HIV through high-risk heterosexual contact and 25 percent acquired HIV through injection drug use. Unfortunately, there are a number of misconceptions regarding HIV transmission among Latinos, including the idea that it can be contracted from mosquitoes and casual forms of contact. Equally unfortunate is the fact that sexuality is usually not discussed openly within the Latino culture, which makes it difficult to implement successful prevention programs. Clearly, in dealing with sexuality, cultural sensitivity is especially important.

Estrada compared and contrasted the sexual risk behaviors of Puerto Rican and Mexican American drug injectors.[33] The behaviors under study included the participant's history of STDs, number of sexual partners, and frequency of condom use. No differences were found between the number of sexual partners Mexican Americans had and the number of sexual partners Puerto Ricans had.[34] As table 5 shows, slightly more Mexican Americans were at immediate risk than Puerto Ricans. Ernie, who works with Latino men in Tucson, Arizona, describes the common Mexican American attitude about sex and HIV:

> The more [power] you have sexually, the more machista you are, the most satisfied you are with being the macho, the image of *el hombre*. But . . . there's also that part where you are at risk of either being infected or not knowing that you are infected and infecting others. And many of these men, they downplay having to use condoms for safe sex or [say] that they don't want to get tested because they are not in that group of people who do get HIV, and that's . . . one of the attitudes of our people, "If I'm not a drug user or if I'm not gay, I can't get the disease because I'm a man and I'm married and that's how it is." (Ernie P., 40)

Table 5. Sexual Risk Behaviors of Two Latino Subgroups

	PUERTO RICAN (%)	MEXICAN AMERICAN (%)
History of STD(s)	29	18
Always use condom	14	7
Sexual risk index rating:		
Low risk	58	47
Intermediate risk	18	24
High risk	24	29

Source: A. L. Estrada, "Drug Use and HIV Risks among African American, Mexican American, and Puerto Rican Drug Injectors," *Journal of Psychoactive Drugs* 30, no. 3 (1998): 247–53.

Estrada and colleagues examined the cultural concept of machismo within the drug-using subculture of Mexican-origin IDUs with intentions to reduce risk behaviors conducive to the transmission of HIV/AIDS. The findings suggest that those Mexican-origin IDUs who have strong machista attitudes are significantly less likely to engage in both sexual and needle risk reduction behaviors.[35]

Risk Factors for Chronic Disease

By and large, the prevalence of risk factors for the major chronic diseases discussed previously are lower among Mexican Americans than among non-Latino whites. Mexican Americans have lower serum cholesterol levels, a lower prevalence of cigarette smoking, and a lower prevalence of hypertension than do non-Latino whites. The only exception is obesity. Approximately 74.8 percent of Mexican American men are overweight or obese in comparison to 72.4 percent of non-Latino white men. Similarly, approximately 73 percent of Mexican American women are overweight or obese in comparison to 57.5 percent of non-Latina white women. There is no question that the lower prevalence of key risk factors for heart disease, stroke, and cancer contribute to the lower mortality rates for these diseases among Mexican Americans in comparison to non-Latino whites. The exception of above-average weight and low glucose tolerance and its contribution to the development of NIDDM continues to be a major cause for concern.

The prevalence of risk factors contributing to HIV disease among Mexican Americans and non-Latino white drug injectors has been examined. Estrada showed that Mexican American drug injectors injected less frequently but disinfected their syringes less often and shared drug paraphernalia more often than did Puerto Ricans or African Americans. Condom use was almost nonexistent among this population. Additionally, a study examining HIV risk behaviors among Mexican-origin gay/bisexual males showed very high rates of unprotected sexual intercourse in combination with drug or alcohol use.[36]

Mexican American Women

The menopause has brought on some problems that I'm faced with, that is the hot flashes, which are not pleasant. I have mild headaches when I don't take my hormonal dose. I get very bloated with water retention, which is very uncomfortable. . . . You also get very lethargic, as far as energy is concerned, unless you start taking your hormone supplements. (Gracie S., 46)

Some of the health issues affecting the lives of Mexican-origin women have already been mentioned. In this section we will highlight three additional issues: fertility patterns, prenatal care, and IPV.

The increase in the U.S. Mexican-origin population is primarily due to two factors: immigration and fertility rates. Among all Latino subgroups in the United States, Mexican American women have the highest **birth rates** and fertility rates. Mexican American women have a birth rate of 24.9 per 1,000 compared to 12.5 per 1,000 for non-Latinos. Further, the fertility rate of Mexican American women was 106.8 per 1,000 compared to 60.5 per 1,000 for non-Latinas.[37] Moreover, Mexican-origin women continue to have children well beyond what is typically referred to as the childbearing years (twenty to thirty-five years of age). These trends suggest a greater need for adequate maternal and child health services.

The age, educational level, and marital status of Mexican American women are important factors in determining the future welfare of both mothers and children. It is well known that Mexican Americans are generally younger than other Latino subgroups and non-Latinos and that their educational attainment levels are lower. Birth data from a National Vital Statistics Report found that 15.3 percent of births of Mexican American women were to those under the age of twenty in comparison to only 7.4 percent for non-Latino whites.[38] We continue to see a similar disparity in the number of births to unmarried women: 45.2 percent of births were to unmarried Mexican American women in comparison to only 24.5 percent to non-Latina white women. These trends suggest increased fertility as well as a potential increase in the "feminization of poverty," in that more Mexican American women become single heads of household.

Appropriate prenatal care is very important to insure the health of both the developing fetus and the expectant mother. Early prenatal care can alert parents and physicians to the possibility of birth defects. Several factors contribute to the use of prenatal care: educational level, income, place of birth, and access to health care. Recent data show that Latina women tend to access and receive prenatal care at a lower rate than do non-Latino whites. In the first trimester (the first three months of pregnancy), 87.9 percent of non-Latina white women received prenatal care compared to

73.7 percent of Latina women. Clearly, more needs to be done to increase prenatal care among Latina women.

Intimate partner violence (IPV) also affects the lives of many Latina women. Data is limited on the prevalence of IPV, and even reported figures could have an underreporting bias. In 1985, the National Family Violence Resurvey found that 17.3 percent of Latino families experienced husband-to-wife violence in the year preceding the survey.[39] In 2000, the National Violence Against Women Survey found that slightly more than 1 out of 5 Latinas reported physical assault.[40] More recent studies have reported life-time and past-year rates among Latinas between 33 and 35 percent.[41] Data derived from the Behavioral Risk Factor Surveillance System compared rates of IPV among Latinas and non-Latina women. Results showed that Latinas reported a lifetime rate of 44.6 percent, compared to 44 percent for non-Latinas.[42] Recent studies suggest that IPV rates are relatively high among Mexican-origin women. For example, Hazen and Soriano (2007) found relatively high rates of IPV. Of the 292 Latina women interviewed, 33.9 percent reported physical violence, 20.9 percent reported sexual coercion, and 82.5 percent reported psychological abuse. Nevertheless, most studies find that the incidence of IPV is similar between Latinas and non-Latina women.

Common types of injuries resulting from this violence include contusions, abrasions, and minor lacerations; fractures or sprains; and repeated chronic injuries. The stress of IPV may also cause psychiatric problems including depression, suicide attempts, feelings of isolation and an inability to cope, posttraumatic stress disorder, and alcohol or drug abuse.[43] Obviously, the most detrimental potential result of intimate partner violence is the death of the abused person.

Several domains contributing to IPV have been identified in the literature.[44] The **etiology** of IPV includes the male's need for power and control, lack of self-esteem, poor impulse control, dysfunctional family patterns, and rigid sex-role expectations (**la sufrida**, *la mártir* [martyr], marianismo, machismo). Other sociocultural factors associated with IPV include acculturation level, underemployment, undereducation, economic stress, and the effects of the Latino male's experience of colonization, poverty, subordination, and exploitation.

Intimate partner violence is a cyclical process. Stress builds up in the male, who is unable to release it in appropriate ways, which then leads to aggression, then remorse. This cycle is often repeated indefinitely. More programs that intervene and stop this cycle of violence are needed.

Agricultural Workers

Mexican Americans are overrepresented in hazardous occupations. One of the most hazardous jobs that leads to increased morbidity and mortality is agricultural work. Such workers encounter five major health-related problems: accidents, pesticide-related illnesses, heat-related illnesses, musculoskeletal disorders, and communicable diseases.[45]

Machinery and farm vehicular accidents are the leading causes of death, injury, and traumatic amputation among agricultural workers. Nevertheless, specific information relating to Mexican-origin agricultural workers is sparse. What is known is that accidents are generally underreported. Most accidents happen during transportation to the fields or in the fields themselves. For example, it is not uncommon for agricultural workers to mistakenly cut off a finger while picking produce, given the monetary incentives to reap the harvest quickly. Agricultural workers who are unable to read English or Spanish frequently use machinery improperly, which can lead to devastating accidents.

Pesticide-related illnesses are a primary cause for concern, since pesticide poisoning affects not only the person exposed but also persons with whom the individual will come into contact, including the unborn. Pesticides are readily absorbed through the lungs, mouth, and skin. Exposure to pesticides may be direct or indirect. Direct exposure occurs through applying pesticides, entering a field where pesticides were recently sprayed, drift of pesticides from one field to an adjacent field, or contact with dry pesticide residue on produce. Indirect exposure may result from eating newly harvested fruits or vegetables without first washing them, eating or smoking with unwashed hands, and drinking from or bathing in runoff from agricultural fields or from barrels initially used for pesticides and then converted into water containers. Pesticide poisoning has short- and long-term effects. Dermatitis, skin inflammation, and rashes are all common symptoms of direct pesticide exposure. Long-term exposure may lead to hematological (blood-system) cancers such as leukemia, Hodgkin's disease, and multiple myeloma. Effects may also occur in utero (in the womb), which increases the chance of damage to the developing fetus and thereby may result in birth defects.

Heat-related illnesses include heat stroke and heat exhaustion, which primarily result from severe dehydration and the lack of protective clothing. Again, due to the pressure to perform, agricultural workers may feel reluctant to take the time out to drink sufficient water. Additionally, most of the work done in the fields is accomplished during the day, with full exposure to the sun. Without proper clothing or protection from the sun, workers can become overheated, resulting in heat stroke and heat exhaustion.

Musculoskeletal problems are a primary cause of physical impairment and activity limitation. Due to the type of work performed, many agricultural workers face long days of constant bending, stooping, kneeling, and heavy lifting. In addition, the now outlawed practice of using the short-handled hoe (called the *mano del Diablo*, or "hand of the devil") contributed to the increase in lower-back problems and disability through constant stooping and bending.

There are at least three types of communicable diseases that affect agricultural workers: bacterial infections, parasitic infections, and viral infections. Among the bacterial infections, salmonellosis and shigellosis are probably the most common. These diseases are a direct result of poor sanitation in the fields or in dwellings. Parasitic diseases resulting from poor sanitary conditions, such as amebiasis, giardiasis, and *Ascaris lumbricoides*, also disproportionately affect agricultural workers and their families. Among the viral infections, hepatitis A, transmitted through poor sanitation and hygiene, can lead to liver problems and disability.

The Mexican American Morbidity and Mortality Paradox

The socioeconomic status of Mexican Americans is lower than that of non-Latino whites and comparable to that of African Americans. Yet researchers have noted what they term the morbidity-mortality paradox among Mexican Americans. With the exception of NIDDM, Mexican Americans generally have lower disease prevalence and disease mortality than do non-Latino whites and blacks despite their socioeconomic disadvantages. In a more recent literature review, Latinos were found to have a significant mortality advantage compared to non-Latino whites and non-Latino blacks.[46]

Several hypotheses have been advanced to explain this paradox, but the two most common are the **salmon bias hypothesis** and the **healthy migrant**

hypothesis. The salmon bias hypothesis states that Mexican Americans who may be near death return to Mexico out of a desire to die in their birthplace. Because these deaths are not accounted for in U.S. mortality statistics, these persons are said to be "statistically immortal," contributing to a lower apparent death rate among Mexican Americans. The healthy migrant hypothesis states that those Mexican Americans in the United States who emigrated from Mexico were generally healthier to begin with. Some researchers have also suggested that there are protective factors present in Mexican American culture that allow some degree of resistance to disease and death. Clearly, more research is needed to fully address the issues raised by this epidemiological paradox.

Several strategies need to be pursued to ameliorate the poor health status of Mexican Americans. These include improving health-care access through greater financial access and through improving the quality of services. Better data are needed to assess health needs and outcomes so as to inform policymakers at all levels of government. More Latino health-care professionals are needed to assist in the development of culturally and linguistically competent health-care programs for the Mexican-origin population. Both private and public partnerships are necessary for the development of proven models to support health promotion and disease prevention within the Mexican-origin community. Clearly, such a shared vision is required if we are to close the gap in health-care resources and improve the health of the Mexican-origin community in the United States.

Concluding Thoughts

This chapter has highlighted key health issues facing the Mexican-origin community as framed within the historical context of health and disease. In traditional indigenous Mesoamerican culture, a person's health depends on the forces of multiple souls in that individual and the balance among these souls. The impact of the Spaniards on the Americas was profound and influenced or changed every aspect of the native cultures, including concepts of health, disease, and medicine. Combined legacies of the indigenous and Spanish cultures provide an important dimension for understanding health and disease in the Mexican-origin community. These early roots, coupled with the contemporary location of Mexican Americans within U.S. society, provide a framework that we can use to better understand the health status of this population. Understanding the cultural dimensions involved in health and medicine can help us in forming strategies to address the health problems this community faces.

Effective strategies can be developed only with an understanding of the age- and gender-specific disease patterns this population faces. For example, as a group, Mexican American children are seriously underimmunized against communicable diseases and infections. Other issues central to this age group, such as obesity and poor dental health, are related to poor diet and poverty. Mexican American adolescents are plagued with health problems such as NIDDM, homicide, and suicide. Moreover, young Mexican American/Chicanas experience early sexual activity and teen pregnancy.

Mexican-origin adults also encounter a higher incidence and prevalence of NIDDM. Complications resulting from late diagnosis and poor medical management of NIDDM are also more prevalent within the Mexican American community than within the non-Latino white community. Other diseases affecting Mexican Americans include cancer, which is the second leading cause of death among Latinos. A key strategy in lowering the incidence and prevalence of breast cancer and cervical cancer, the most common cancers among Mexican American women, is early detection and screening. Unfortunately, in practice, the development of culturally and linguistically sensitive outreach and information programs about preventative services is still emerging in health-care settings. The use of *promotoras* (community health workers) to improve health education on these topics is a strategy that shows promise in providing greater awareness and access to these important health programs. Model programs must be developed and evaluated for their ability to enhance the health status of this growing community. Future research on Mexican American women's health should focus on the underutilization of prenatal care and the extent of IPV.

Finally, occupational location, the type and economic sector of a person's employment, is a major influence on health-related injuries and diseases. This chapter focused on agricultural workers as an important subcategory of Mexican-origin people who are at greater health risk because of the work they perform. It is well established in the literature that farmworkers are more vulnerable to musculoskeletal diseases and pesticide poisoning as a result of their jobs. The unique occupational position of these workers requires additional sensitivity in the screening and treatment of diseases. An important phenomenon that needs further study is the Mexican

American morbidity and mortality paradox. Mexican Americans appear to have lower disease prevalence and disease mortality than non-Latinos with similar socioeconomic characteristics. We must determine whether this is a result of cultural protective factors, physical characteristics, or simply inaccurate data.

Discussion Exercises

1. Discuss the origins of cultural beliefs about health and disease based on Aztec and European/Spanish concepts of medicine.

2. How does socioeconomic status affect the health status of Mexican Americans?

3. How do Mexican cultural beliefs and attitudes (machismo, marianismo, familismo, personalismo, etc.) influence the help-seeking behaviors and attitudes about health within the Mexican-origin population? What role does acculturation play in decisions regarding health?

4. Explain how the terms "incidence," "prevalence," "relative risk," and "attributable risk" are useful in designing disease-prevention programs for the Mexican-origin community.

5. Discuss the three levels of disease prevention and give one example of each.

6. What factors affect the health status of Mexican American children? What are the major health issues facing this group? What issues emerge as these children progress through adolescence into adulthood?

7. Name some of the risk factors that can be modified to reduce the chance of diabetes, heart disease, and cancer.

8. How are Mexican American women affected by the issues of fertility patterns, prenatal care, and IPV? How do cultural beliefs and gender roles influence women's health decisions regarding these issues?

9. Discuss the reasons why Mexican-origin workers are disproportionately exposed to work-related environmental and safety hazards. What are some of the conditions that can result from this exposure?

10. What are some recommendations for improving the health status of Mexican Americans and Latinos in general in the years to come? What would you recommend based on the information in this chapter?

Notes

1. Mesoamerica refers to the area extending from central Mexico south and east through northern Central America.

2. B. R. Ortiz de Montellano, *Aztec Medicine, Health, and Nutrition* (New Brunswick, NJ: Rutgers University Press, 1990).

3. I. Cuellar, B. Arnold, and R. Moldonado, "Acculturation Rating Scale for Mexican Americans—II: A Revision of the Original ARSMA Scale," *Hispanic Journal of Behavioral Sciences* 17, no. 3 (1995): 275–304; see also C. Negy and D. J. Woods, "The Importance of Acculturation in Understanding Research with Hispanic Americans," *Hispanic Journal of Behavioral Sciences* 14, no. 2 (1992): 224–47.

4. K. S. Markides, D. J. Lee, and L. A. Ray, "Acculturation and Hypertension in Mexican Americans," *Ethnicity and Disease* 3, no. 1 (1993): 70–74; J. Sundquist and M. A. Winkleby, "Cardiovascular Risk Factors in Mexican American Adults: A Transcultural Analysis of NHANES III, 1988–1994," *American Journal of Public Health* 89, no. 5 (1999): 723–30; J. M. Flack et al., "Epidemiology of Minority Health," *Health Psychology* 14, no. 7 (1995): 592–600.

5. H. C. Triandas, *The Analysis of Subjective Culture* (New York: John Wiley, 1972).

6. R. Vargas and S. Martínez, *Razalogía: Community Learning for a New Society* (Oakland, CA: Razagente Associates, 1984).

7. S. J. Andrade and C. Doria-Ortiz, "Nuestro Bienestar: A Mexican-American Community-Based Definition of Health Promotion in the Southwestern United States," *Drugs, Education, Prevention, and Policy* 2, no. 2 (1995): 129–45. Emphasis in original.

8. P. Freire, *Pedagogy of the Oppressed* (New York: Continuum, 1995).

9. D. Altschuler, G. Strangler, K. Berkley, and L. Burton, "Supporting Youth in Transition to Adulthood: Lessons Learned from Child Welfare and Juvenile Justice," Center for Juvenile Justice Reform, 2009.

10. H. Rodríguez-Trias and A. B. Ramírez de Arellano, "The Health of Children and Youth," in *Latino Health in the United States: A Growing Challenge*, ed. M. Aguirre-Molina and C. W. Molina, 115–33 (Washington, DC: American Public Health Association, 1994).

11. American Community Survey, S0201, "Selected Population Profile in the United States," in *2009 American Community Survey 1-Year Estimates*, 2010.

12. J. Kominski, T. A. Kominski, and R. A. Kominski, "Education and Synthetic Work-Life Earnings Estimates," *American Community Survey Reports*, ACS-14 (Washington DC: U.S. Census Bureau, 2011).

13. Centers for Disease Control and Prevention, *Vaccines and Immunizations, Statistics and Surveillance: 2009 Table Data*, retrieved November 3, 2010, from http://www.cdc.gov/.

14. P. J. Gergen, T. Ezzati, and H. Russell, "DTP Immunization Status and Tetanus Antitoxin Status of Mexican American Children Ages Six Months through Eleven Years," *American Journal of Public Health* 78 (1988): 1446–50.

15. Centers for Disease Control and Prevention, *NCHS Health E-Stat, Prevalence of Obesity among Children and Adolescents: United States Trends, 1963–1965 Through 2007–2008*, retrieved on November 4, 2010, from http://www.cdc.gov.

16. B. A. Dye et al., "Trends in Oral Health Status: United States, 1988–1994 and 1999–2004," National Center for Health Statistics, *Vital Health Statistics* 11, no. 248 (2007): 1–92.

17. H. S. Glaser and K. L. Jones, "Non-insulin Dependent Diabetes Mellitus in Mexican American Children," *Western Journal of Medicine* 168, no. 1 (1998): 11–16.

18. D. Neufeld et al., "Early Presentation of Type 2 Diabetes in Mexican American Youth," *Diabetes Care* 21 (1998): 80–86.

19. A. de la Torre, "Health: Current Issues and Trends," in *Latinas in the United States: A Historical Encyclopedia*, ed. V. L. Ruiz and V. S. Korrol, 311 (Bloomington: Indiana University Press, 2006).

20. National Adolescent Health Information Center, *National Data Project: Homicide Mortality*, retrieved November 28, 2010, from http://nahic.ucsf.edu/.

21. Centers for Disease Control and Prevention, *Suicide: Facts at a Glance*, Summer 2009, retrieved on November 5, 2010, from http://www.cdc.gov/.

22. American Diabetes Association, *Diabetes Statistics*, retrieved on November 5, 2010, from http://www.diabetes.org/.

23. M. Harris et al., "Prevalence of Diabetes, Impaired Fasting Glucose, and Impaired Glucose Tolerance in U.S. Adults: The Third National Health and Nutrition Examination Survey, 1988–1994," *Diabetes Care* 21 (1998): 518–24.

24. Centers for Disease Control and Prevention, "Differences in Prevalence of Obesity among Black, White, and Hispanic Adults—United States, 2006–2008," *Mortality and Morbidity Weekly Report* (July 17, 2009).

25. Centers for Disease Control and Prevention, "National Diabetes Fact Sheet: National Estimates and General Information on Diabetes and Prediabetes in the United States, 2011" (Atlanta, GA: U.S. Department of Health and Human Services, Centers for Disease Control and Prevention, 2011).

26. S. M. Haffner et al., "Role of Obesity and Fat Distribution in Non-insulin Dependent Diabetes Mellitus in Mexican Americans and Non-Hispanic Whites," *Diabetes Care* 9 (1986): 153–61; E. J. Boyko et al., "Higher Insulin and C-peptide Concentrations in Hispanic Populations at High Risk for NIDDM: San Luis Valley Diabetes Study," *Diabetes* 40 (1991): 509–15.

27. *Morbidity and Mortality: 2012 Chart Book Cardiovascular, Lung, and Blood Diseases*, National Institutes of Health, National Heart, Lung, and Blood Institute, February 2012.

28. I. Hajjar and T. A. Kotchen, "Trends in Prevalence, Awareness, Treatment and Control of Hypertension in the United States, 1988–2000," *Journal of the American Medical Association* 290 (2003): 199–206.

29. A. S. Go et al., "Heart Disease and Stroke Statistics: 2013 Update; A Report from the American Heart Association," *Circulation* 127 (2013): e6–e245.

30. A. Jemal et al., "Annual Report to the Nation on the Status of Cancer, 1975–2009, Featuring the Burden and Trends in Human Papillomavirus (HPV)-Associated Cancers and HPV Vaccination Levels," *Journal of the National Cancer Institute* 105, no. 3 (February 6, 2013): 175–201.

31. M. Johnson-Kozlow, S. Roussos, L. Rovniak, and M. Hovell, "Colorectal Cancer Test Use among Californians of Mexican Origin: Influence of Language Barriers," *Ethnicity & Disease* 19, no. 3 (2009): 315–22; M. Johnson-Kozlow, "Colorectal Cancer Screening of Californian Adults of Mexican Origin as a Function of Acculturation," *Journal of Immigrant and Minority Health* 12 (2010): 454–61.

32. Centers for Disease Control and Prevention. *HIV Surveillance Report, 2011*, vol. 23, retrieved on December 5, 2013, from http://www.cdc.gov.

33. A. L. Estrada, "Drug Use and HIV Risks among African American, Mexican American, and Puerto Rican Drug Injectors," *Journal of Psychoactive Drugs* 30, no. 3 (1998): 247–53.

34. Ibid.

35. A. L. Estrada, B. D. Estrada, and G. Quintero, "The Influence of Cultural Values on Self-Efficacy in Reducing HIV Risk Behaviors," Mexican American Studies and Research Center, Working Paper Series no. 28, September 1999.

36. A. L. Estrada, "HIV Risk Behaviors among Gay Latinos Residing in the U.S.-Mexico Border Area." Paper presented to the 120th Annual Meeting of the American Public Health Association, Washington, DC, April 1992.

37. J. A. Martin et al., "Births: Final data for 2004," *National Vital Statistics Reports* 55, no. 1 (Hyattsville, MD: National Center for Health Statistics, 2006).

38. Ibid.

39. M. A. Straus and C. Smith, "Violence in Hispanic Families in the United States: Incidence Rates and Structural Interpretations," in *Physical Violence in American Families: Risk Factors and Adaptations to Violence in 8,145 Families*, ed. M. A. Straus and R. J. Gelles, 341–67 (New Brunswick, NJ: Transaction, 1990).

40. P. Tjaden and N. Thoennes, "Extent, Nature, and Consequences of Intimate Partner Violence: Findings from the National Violence Against Women Survey." (Washington, DC: U.S. Department of Justice, 2000).

41. A. L. Hazen and F. I. Soriano, "Experiences with Intimate Partner Violence among Latina Women," *Violence Against Women* 13 (2007): 562. A. E. Bonomi et al., "Intimate Partner Violence in Latina and Non-Latina Women," *American Journal of Preventive Medicine* 36, no. 1 (2009): 43–48.

42. Centers for Disease Control and Prevention, "Adverse Health Conditions and Health Risk Behaviors Associated with Intimate Partner Violence: United States, 2005," *Morbidity and Mortality Weekly Report* 57 (2008): 113–17.

43. K. Fedovskiy, S. Higgins, and A. Paranjape, "Intimate Partner Violence: How Does It Impact Major Depressive Disorder and Post Traumatic Stress Disorder among Immigrant Latinas?" *Journal of Immigrant and Minority Health* 10 (2008): 45–51.

44. M. M. Zambrana, *Mejor Sola que Mal Acompañada: For the Latina in an Abusive Relationship* (Seattle: The Seal Press, 1985).

45. G. Friedman-Jiménez and J. S. Ortiz, "Occupational Health," in *Latino Health in the United States: A Growing Challenge*, ed. C. W. Molina and M. Aguirre-Molina, 341–89 (Washington, DC: American Public Health Association, 1994).

46. J. M. Ruiz, P. Steffen, and T. B. Smith, "The Hispanic Mortality Paradox: A Systematic Review and Meta-analysis of the Longitudinal Literature," *American Journal of Public Health* 103 (2013): e1–e9.

Suggested Readings

Adams, D. L. *Health Issues for Women of Color: A Cultural Diversity Perspective.* Thousand Oaks, CA: Sage Publications, 1995.

Delgado, J. L. *Salud! A Latina's Guide to Total Health—Body, Mind, and Spirit.* New York: HarperCollins, 1997.

Furino, A. *Health Policy and the Hispanic.* Boulder, CO: Westview Press, 1992.

Molina, C. W., and M. Aguirre-Molina, eds. *Latino Health in the U.S.: A Growing Challenge.* Washington, DC: American Public Health Association, 1994.

National Center for Health Statistics. *Health, United States, 1998 (with Socioeconomic Status and Health Chartbook).* Hyattsville, MD: U.S. Department of Health and Human Services, 1998.

The Office of Minority Health Resource Center website: http://www.minorityhealth .hhs.gov/.

Plepys, C. *Health Status Indicators: Differentials by Race and Hispanic Origin.* Hyattsville, MD: U.S. Department of Health and Human Services, 1995.

Qunitero, G. A., and A. L. Estrada. "Cultural Models of Masculinity and Drug Use: 'Machismo,' Heroin, and Street Survival on the U.S.-Mexico Border." *Contemporary Drug Problems* 25 (1998): 147–68.

Chapter 3

Understanding Substance Abuse and AIDS

"One Starts with Marijuana"

The **co-occurrence** of substance use, violence, and HIV/AIDS risk behaviors poses serious problems for the Latino community. In this chapter we will examine several topics: (1) the **epidemiology** (patterns) of substance use among Latino adolescents and adults; (2) the available evidence on the cause of substance use; (3) the co-occurrence of substance abuse with violence and HIV/AIDS; and (4) issues related to the prevention of substance abuse among youth and adolescents.

The **syndemic** of substance abuse, HIV/AIDS, and violence are cause for particular concern among Latinos.[1] According to the CDC, in 2011 injection drug use accounted for 8 percent of diagnosed HIV infections among Latino male adults and adolescents, and 14 percent of diagnosed HIV infections among Latina female adults and adolescents.[2] However, to address substance abuse, violence, and HIV/AIDS prevention for Latinos, it becomes very important to differentiate **epidemiological patterns** associated with increased risk among the various Latino subgroups (Puerto Rican, Cuban, Central or South American, Mexican American). These Latino subgroups may exhibit different drug-use patterns, and understanding such differences can maximize the chances for successful substance-abuse treatment and HIV/AIDS prevention programs.

Few national databases on substance abuse or HIV/AIDS differentiate among the major Latino subgroups. This lack of differentiation has resulted in the spread of many substance abuse and HIV/AIDS prevention strategies that are too generic to be meaningful. We must ask ourselves whether it continues to make sense to implement prevention models that do not incorporate key cultural elements related to behavioral change of the minority groups with whom we work. Do cultural prevention models have greater impact on reducing substance abuse, violence, or HIV/AIDS than do generic models? Would prevention resources be better used if the **epidemiological profiles** of Latino subgroups were matched to primary, secondary, and tertiary prevention efforts? Are cultural models of prevention more cost-effective than generic models? These questions, and others, need to be addressed if we wish to be truly responsive to the heartfelt needs of people living with and dying from the adverse health consequences of drug use.

Prevalence of Drug Use among Latino Adolescents and Adults

> Once one is involved in drugs, bad company follows, problems, jail, etc., etc., fights, violence. This is what drugs bring into one's life and nothing else. That is what I believe because I have gone through it so much, and I would not want today's youth to fall into the clutches of vice. It would make me very happy that they would listen to me and that they would attend to my words. (Enrique A., 30)

Since large national databases usually do not differentiate among Latino subgroups, the data available can only provide a picture of substance-abuse trends among Latinos in general. The epidemiology of substance abuse among Latino adolescents can be assessed through existing databases and research findings. The findings of sources such as the Youth Risk Behavior Survey,[3] the Monitoring the Future Study,[4] the National Household Survey on Drug Abuse,[5] the Hispanic Community Health Study/Study of Latinos,[6] and the Hispanic Health and Nutrition Examination Survey[7] (HHANES) are particularly relevant.

Latino Adolescents

> [W]hen I was at Edison Elementary School . . . my friends were already using drugs. I chose [marijuana] because it was available. From there [I] tried pills, cocaine, and, well, in school, as a youth, one does not know how to say no. One starts with marijuana, then cocaine followed by heroin, ending with more dangerous substances. (Enrique A., 30)

Among both males and females enrolled in high school, lifetime use of (that is, whether one has ever used) alcohol, marijuana, and cocaine was higher for Latino youth than for other racial and ethnic groups. For youth in high school, Latino males and females had higher rates than both African Americans and non-Latino whites for lifetime use of alcohol and cocaine; however, they had lower lifetime prevalence rates for marijuana. These trends suggest that drug use in Latino communities begins early and continues well into the late teen years at higher rates than in African American and non-Latino white communities.

Latino Adults

> I believe that once you are an alcoholic or an addict, you are always an alcoholic or an addict, and you have to be careful of backsliding. (Danny F., 36)

In 2009, the Substance Abuse and Mental Health Services Administration (SAMHSA) examined the use of alcohol, tobacco, and illicit drugs among the U.S. population aged twelve and older.[8] The survey noted several trends:

- Almost 8 percent of the adult Latino population currently engages in illicit drug use.
- Latinos had the highest rate of binge drinking of all the racial groups (25 percent).
- Latinos had a higher substance-abuse rate than both non-Latino whites and African Americans (10.1 percent in comparison to 9 percent and 8.8 percent, respectively).
- The most commonly used illicit drug was marijuana (76.6 percent).

These data suggest that the primary drug of choice for Latino adults is marijuana, with the use of other illegal drugs occurring at much lower rates. Overall, Latinos had higher illegal drug use than did non-Latino whites. Although information specific to the various Latino subgroups is not easily attained, one study sheds light on key differences and patterns among the major Latino subgroups. Conducted jointly by the Substance Abuse and Mental Health Services Administration (SAMHSA), Office of Applied Studies (OAS), and National Opinion Research Center, the *Prevalence of Substance Use among Racial and Ethnic Subgroups in the U.S.* report examined the patterns of substance use among different ethnicities, including Cubans, Mexicans, Puerto Ricans, and other Latinos.[9] Among those of Mexican or Puerto Rican origin or descent, male English speakers between the ages of eighteen and twenty-five had the highest marijuana use rates. Subgroup differences were observed with relation to cocaine use as well, with individuals between the ages of eighteen and thirty-four being two to seven times more likely than those of other age groups to have used cocaine. More men reported use than did women, as well as more English speakers than Spanish speakers. Overall, the subgroup with the highest reported rate of cocaine use was Mexican Americans. Puerto Ricans had the highest prevalence of illicit drug use in the past year (13.3 percent), with Mexicans trailing right behind (12.7 percent).

Injection Drug Use among Mexican Americans

The "hidden" nature of the drug-injecting population makes accurate estimates difficult; however, a National Survey on Drug Use and Health (NSDUH) report estimated that there were an average of 425,000 IDUs in the United States.[10] Latinos and other minority groups are probably overrepresented in this group, yet surprisingly little is known about the prevalence of injection drug use and associated risks among Latinos in general and Mexican Americans in particular. Data collected as part of the household survey of the National Institute on Drug Abuse (NIDA) show only a 2.2 percent prevalence rate for any use of needles among Mexican Americans.[11]

Casual Factors in Substance Use

Several causal factors are reported in the substance-abuse literature. These factors fall into three broad areas: social context, individual/interpersonal factors, and acculturation.

Social Context and Initiation of Substance Use

Factors considered in the area of social context include laws and norms favorable to substance use, availability of legal and illegal drugs, low socio-economic status, unemployment, crime, and poverty levels in particular neighborhoods.

Laws and social or cultural norms that are favorable toward drug use are considered to be modifiable risk factors; that is, they are amenable to change. Even though laws related to age of purchase for tobacco and alcohol exist in many states, youth can still obtain these substances relatively easily through falsified identification or by having older individuals, including parents, purchase these products for them. Norms favoring the use of certain substances are also prevalent. For example, it is not uncommon for parents to purchase alcohol for their children to drink at their own parties with parental supervision. This act sends a message that alcohol consumption is okay if conducted under parental supervision. Norms among youth also tend to encourage consumption of both alcohol and illegal drugs.

> I used street drugs. . . . I think smoking weed and drinking a little bit of beer was like a daily thing. (Danny F., 36)

Availability of both legal and illegal drugs is another important factor contributing to use. Many studies have shown that when drugs are available, use tends to increase.[12] Perceived availability of drugs is correlated with age and grade level of students, with older students in higher grades having higher rates of use and greater perceived availability.

Typically, those who live at or below the federal poverty level also live in neighborhoods where there is a high prevalence of crime, including drug dealing and drug use. Since Mexican Americans and other Latino subgroups tend to reside in neighborhoods (*barrios*) where these factors coexist, it is not surprising that consumption of both legal and illegal drugs tends to be higher.

Individual and Interpersonal Factors in the Initiation of Substance Use

> A lot of my friends started using and I never wanted to use. Little by little they came up . . . [to me] telling me that they started getting high. One of the major things is that I always wanted to identify with something and ever since I was nine years old, I started getting lost, like where's my place. (Danny F., 36)

Factors related to drug use include poor family management, association with drug-using peers, early onset of drug use, and antisocial behavior. Family management issues include lack of clear expectations for behavior, lack of monitoring, lack of caring, and inconsistent or excessively severe discipline. These are significantly correlated with the initiation and maintenance of substance use. For example, a study of in-school youth in the Arizona-Sonora border area found that more than one-third of 10th graders were allowed to stay out past 10:00 p.m. during school nights, and more than 50 percent were allowed to stay out past midnight on weekends.[13] Such lack of parental monitoring can easily lead to substance use among youth.

Other studies have shown that association with drug-using peers is highly correlated with substance use and that peer pressure to use both legal and illegal drugs is not uncommon.

Among Latino, African American, and non-Latino white 12th graders, 55 percent thought that their close friends would disapprove of them experimenting (trying once or twice) with marijuana, and 74 percent reported that their friends would disapprove of them smoking marijuana regularly. However, according to recent evidence from the Monitoring the Future Study, Latinos in 8th and 10th grade report higher rates of any illicit drug use than do both African Americans and non-Latino whites; however, Latinos in 12th grade report lower illicit drug use rates than non-Latino whites but higher rates than African Americans. This same observation holds for marijuana, inhalants, Ecstasy (MDMA), cocaine, and heroin use. Latino 8th, 10th, and 12th graders report higher use of crack cocaine than do their African American and non-Latino white counterparts. This trend is accompanied by a similar increase in reported use of substances among friends. This relationship reflects several different patterns: a person with friends who use a drug will be more likely to try that drug, a person who is already using a drug will be more likely to introduce friends to the experience, and users are more likely to establish friendships with other users.[14] Peer approval of drug use is also correlated with the initiation and maintenance of drug use. The study of in-school youth in the Arizona-Sonora border region found that 23 percent of 10th graders' friends would approve of alcohol use and 15 percent would approve of marijuana use.[15]

The early onset of substance use is also associated with the maintenance of substance use behaviors. A 2003 report by NIDA shows the age of first use of cigarettes, alcohol, and marijuana for youth as falling between twelve and seventeen.[16] Between 1991 and 1998, Latino youth initiated cigarette smoking on average at twelve and a half years of age compared to twelve years of age for African American and non-Latino white youth. Latino youth initiated alcohol use at a slightly older age than non-Latino whites but a younger age than African Americans. Latino youth initiated marijuana use at a slightly younger age that non-Latino white and African American youth, at thirteen and a half years of age compared to fourteen years of age.

Antisocial behavior is also highly correlated with substance use, as shown in table 6. Although the percentages of antisocial behavior accompanying marijuana use are high, the percentage increases with cocaine use in the

Table 6. Correlation of Antisocial Behavior with Drug Use among Adolescents

DRUG USED IN PAST 30 DAYS	NON-LATINO WHITE		LATINO	
	INVOLVED IN FIGHT* (%)	CARRIED WEAPON† (%)	INVOLVED IN FIGHT* (%)	CARRIED WEAPON† (%)
Marijuana	48.5	24.8	64.8	37.9
Cocaine	59.9	47.3	82.1	54.6
No drug use	31.9	15.1	37.1	16.3

Source: National Institute on Drug Abuse, 2003, *Drug Use Among Racial/Ethnic Minorities* (NIH Publication No. 03-3888), Bethesda, MD.
* In the past year.
† In the past month.

past thirty days.[17] Among youths who had not used drugs within the past month, Latino respondents reported antisocial behavior more frequently than did non-Latino white respondents.

Acculturation and Nativity Factors in the Initiation of Substance Use

When you are drugged up you look for fights at school, you make graffiti, you fight with other members of the gang. It would make us so mad when they would call us "wetbacks." That is why we joined that gang, because we were wetbacks, and as time went by, more wetbacks joined the gang. Being in the company of five or ten friends, all under the influence of drugs, we would beat people to unconsciousness with sticks or whatever you want to call it! (Enrique A., 30)

Some research has shown that acculturation level is correlated with both legal and illegal drug use. Felix-Ortiz and Newcomb suggest that research must extend the concept of acculturation to be more inclusive of cultural identity.[18] For them, cultural identity more accurately represents the process that occurs as part of personality formation among Latino adolescents. They suggest several ways in which cultural identity can affect drug use. It may increase risk for persons who strongly identify as Mexican American because their values and behavior conflict with those of the dominant culture. Conversely, cultural identity may be protective, in that persons who strongly identify with Mexican American culture may be at reduced risk because Mexican American values and behavior do not support the use of drugs. Similarly, bicultural identity may be risk-increasing due to the stress of negotiating two cultures (**acculturative stress**); or, it may be protective due to the adaptive integration of persons who have the skills to negotiate both cultures.[19]

Recent research shows that acculturation level and nativity status are significantly associated with substance use. Latino adults born in the United States have higher past-month rates of alcohol use, binge alcohol use, and illicit drug use than do non-U.S. born Latinos. Borges and colleagues (2011) have convincingly demonstrated that lifetime drug use among the Mexican-origin population significantly increases if one is born in the United States.[20] In another study, Grant and colleagues (2004) found that U.S.-born Mexican Americans, compared to their foreign-born counterparts, were 2.6 times more likely to have any alcohol disorder, 7.5 times more likely to have any drug-use disorder, and 8.6 times more likely to have any drug dependence.

To date, research findings linking acculturation, cultural identity, or acculturative stress to substance use among Latinos have been contradictory. A more extensive examination is needed of the multiple and complex interactions among culture, discrimination and prejudice, and socioeconomic status in relation to substance use.

The Co-occurrence of Violence and Substance Use among Mexican American Adolescents

> My mother . . . left to go take care of her mom when I was fourteen. . . . I never wanted to be in a gang, and I never wanted to use drugs or alcohol. . . . There was substance abuse in my house. There was violence, and it became a hopeless place and a lot of my friends started using and I never wanted to use. (Danny F., 36)

Several studies on violence and substance use have found a high correlation between the two, yet a causal relationship is difficult to establish without **longitudinal data** that follow a group of people over many years. Otherwise, it is difficult to disentangle which came first, drug use or violence. Some research has indicated that the interrelationship between drug use and violence is complex, depending in part on the drug consumed, the personality of the person consuming the drug, and the context in which the two coexist. Clearly, several factors are involved in this relationship, for example, low self-esteem, poor academic performance, and delinquency. Poor academic performance is higher among Latino youth than among other youth. Moreover, Chávez, Edwards, and Oetting found that school dropouts and students with poor academic achievement were more likely to be both perpetrators and victims of violence.[21] Among Mexican American youth in the study, those who were dropouts had higher rates of being beaten by parents or peers, stabbed, or shot than those Mexican American students in good or even poor academic standing.

Adverse Health Consequences of Drug Use

Drug use has serious health consequences, including HIV/AIDS and related risk behaviors, drug-related emergency room episodes, and drug-related deaths.

HIV/AIDS and Related Behaviors

As mentioned previously, in 2011, among Latino men, injection drug use accounted for 8 percent of diagnosed HIV infections, and among Latina women, for 14 percent of diagnosed HIV infections.[22] In the Southwest, where the vast majority of Latinos are of Mexican origin, AIDS rates attributed to injection drug use range from a high of 13.3 percent in Arizona to a low of 6.9 percent in California.[23]

Although examining incidence and prevalence rates is important, attention must also be paid to the **behavioral epidemiology** of HIV risk among Mexican American IDUs. This focus must include many injection and sexual risk behaviors if we are to fully understand activities conducive to HIV transmission and develop appropriate strategies to reduce these risks. Several studies have characterized risk behaviors associated with HIV transmission among IDUs.[24] Briefly, these behaviors include the frequency of drug injection, the frequency and proportion of injection with used needles, the number of needle/syringe-sharing partners, injection with specific drugs such as heroin, cocaine, and heroin mixtures (**speedballs**), and indirect sharing of drug-injection equipment such as **cookers, cotton**, and the **rinse water**.

Within the past decade there has been an increase in research examining HIV risk behaviors in the U.S.-Mexico border area.[25] One of the first was Estrada and colleagues, who reported on the prevalence of HIV risk behaviors in the Southwest in a study comparing border-area Latinos (those residing in Arizona, California, and Texas) with non-border-area Latinos, non-Latino whites, and African Americans. The findings indicated that border-area Latinos were most likely to share needles with two or more persons (74 percent), with non-Latino whites being the next most likely (65 percent), followed by African Americans (59 percent) and non-border-area Latinos (58 percent). Border-area Latinos were less likely than African Americans and non-border-area Latinos to always use a clean needle. Moreover, they were less likely to use bleach (which kills the HIV virus) as a disinfectant than the other three groups. More recent research in the U.S.-Mexico border area suggests high-risk behaviors among IDUs and female sex workers.

In a recent study examining HIV risk behaviors in a sample of Mexican American IDUs in California, Martinez et al. found that this population had concerning rates of distributive and receptive syringe sharing (31 percent and 23 percent, respectively). These rates were similar to their non-Latino white counterparts (29 percent and 26 percent, respectively) but almost twice as high as the rates for African Americans (15 percent and 12 percent, respectively). The study also found that Mexican American IDUs had significantly lower levels of syringe covering (percentage of single use per syringe) than did non-Latino whites and African Americans.[26]

Clearly, given the frequent sharing of injection equipment with others in the drug-using social network, the high frequency of injection, and the general lack of adequate disinfection among Mexican American IDUs, this group is sitting on a time bomb. It is indeed fortunate that the HIV **seroprevalence** is low (on average about 3 percent to 5 percent) among Mexican American drug injectors in the Southwest. The prevalence of hepatitis B and C is very high among IDUs, however. These studies suggest that HIV/AIDS risk-reduction programs should specifically target the needle-using social network of Mexican American injectors.

Among IDUs, risk of HIV transmission via sex remains particularly high.[27] Behaviors to be targeted to reduce HIV risk include frequency of condom use; exchanging sex for money, drugs, or both; and the number of sexual partners who are IDUs. With respect to exchanging sex for money and/or drugs, Mexican American IDUs reported exchanging sex for money or drugs an average of less than once in the last thirty days. However, condom use was found to be almost nonexistent. Additionally, other research with Mexican American IDUs has found that few make the connection between risky needle practices and the risk of HIV transmission to a non-IDU partner through unprotected sex. This connection needs to be made explicit for both the IDU and his or her sexual partner. Moreover, some injection methods, namely **backloading** and **frontloading**, involve sharing syringes rather than needles. Syringe sharing usually occurs with a common or pooled purchase of the injected drug. Because the syringe may become contaminated with blood, syringe sharing is another possible means of HIV transmission. Risk behaviors among Mexican American IDUs are unlikely to change if prevention efforts focus on needle sharing while ignoring syringe sharing and the reasons for doing so and on condom use without making an explicit connection between needle risk and sexual risk.

> The sexual power is also seen in some men who are machistas, that because they are married or have a common-law wife or have a girlfriend, they can also engage in having sex with other men as long as they are not identified as being homosexual, as being a gay individual . . . compounding that with alcohol or any other drug use, the power increases. (Ernie P., 40)

Men who have sex with men and inject drugs pose threats for HIV transmission both among themselves and to others. However, few studies have examined injection drug use among gay men and fewer still have examined this issue among Mexican Americans. Ibañez and colleagues focused on substance abuse, sexual risk, and psychological distress among HIV-positive gay/bisexual men. In their study, they found that a significantly higher percentage of gay men than straight men are IDUs (74.2 percent compared to 25.8 percent).[28]

LATINO YOUTH AND ADOLESCENTS

Several studies have shown that Latino adolescents are among the least informed about HIV/AIDS of all ethnic groups, and they generally have more misconceptions about HIV transmission than do others.[29] Most youth do not perceive themselves to be at risk for HIV infection,[30] nor do they usually change their behaviors as a consequence of HIV information.[31]

Sexuality and sexual knowledge among Latino youth are not well understood, but a few studies have been completed. Norris and Ford examined acculturation, ethnicity, and gender in terms of condom beliefs and found that more acculturated Latino youth were more likely to have positive views about condoms than less acculturated Latino youth.[32] This was highly evident in the belief that a woman who carries a condom is looking for sex. Less acculturated Latino youth were more likely to agree with this statement than were more acculturated Latino youth. The lack of contraceptive knowledge among this population became obvious as the authors were forced to eliminate eleven of their Latino respondents from statistical analyses because they had never heard of or seen a condom in their lives. Further, Moore and Erickson found that Latino students had less factual knowledge about sexuality, particularly birth control, than did African Americans or non-Latino whites.[33] However, these authors found no significant differences between Latinos and other ethnic groups in terms of sexual behavior such as frequency of intercourse, contraception use, pregnancy history, talking about birth control and STDs with partners, and age of first sexual intercourse.

In terms of HIV/AIDS education strategies, most adolescents prefer peer-based strategies that are innovative and that do not "just talk about the same old thing." Most adolescents say they would like an HIV-positive person to talk to them about AIDS and to show them what the disease does to the body. It is difficult for most youth to identify readily with a disease like AIDS that shows no symptoms for a period of many years. Thus, HIV/AIDS prevention among Mexican American youth must be threefold: (1) increasing awareness of sexual behaviors that can lead to HIV/AIDS infection, (2) increasing the understanding that drug use is an HIV risk factor, and (3) reducing HIV risk behaviors currently practiced.

LATINA WOMEN

In general, female IDUs who are in a relationship are likely to be with a man who is also an IDU; conversely, the majority of male IDUs are in primary relationships with women who do not use drugs.[34] Women IDUs are also reported to have more medical problems than their male counterparts, including poor nutrition, repeated infections, and STDs. They also may experience more stress because of responsibility for children, lack of support from family, lack of financial resources, anxiety, and low self-esteem.[35] These women may also turn to prostitution as a means of financial support. Non-injecting women who are in relationships with male IDUs are confronted with similar economic and emotional issues. A major difference, however, is that women who do not inject drugs may not perceive themselves as being at risk, not realizing that a sexual relationship with an

IDU may put them and their future offspring in danger.[36] The failure to recognize such risks is exacerbated in relationships where the male hides his drug use from his spouse or significant other.[37]

There are only a small number of promising interventions that target female sexual partners of IDUs. One is the WHEEL (Women Helping to Empower and Enhance Lives) project, sponsored by NIDA. This intervention focuses on educating such women so that they will become empowered to take responsibility for their own health and safety. Strategies include educating them about their HIV transmission risks, increasing their awareness of and confronting denial, training them in skills necessary for negotiating and practicing safer sex, counseling them in methods of negotiating safer sex practices with their partner(s), and educating them in how to obtain needed resources from community service agencies and advocacy groups. CDC's Prevention Research Synthesis Project has documented several evidence-based interventions specific for Latinas. These include S.A.F.E., CONNECT, Women's Health Promotion, and SEPA (*Salud, Educacion, Prevencion y Autocuidado*). Each of these interventions takes a comprehensive approach to increasing communication about and negotiating safer sex skills, reducing sexual risk behaviors, increasing self-efficacy and self-esteem, and enhancing personal health.

Drug-Related Emergency Room Episodes

Drug-related episodes at hospital emergency rooms provide an important measure of the health risks associated with drug use. Records of these visits indicate increases or decreases in the incidence of problems associated with a particular drug or drug combination. The primary source of data on drug-related emergency room visits is the Drug Abuse Warning Network (DAWN), a large-scale, ongoing data collection system that monitors the adverse consequences of drug abuse as reported by selected hospital emergency rooms and medical examiner's offices in the nation.[38] As shown in table 7, among Latinos the six illicit drugs most frequently mentioned in emergency room visits were cocaine, marijuana, heroin, PCP, Ecstasy (MDMA), and methamphetamines.

In 2011 Latinos represented 10.9 percent of emergency room visits related to illicit drug compared to 58.7 percent for non-Latino whites and 22.3 percent for African Americans. As shown in table 8, Latinos also have the lowest percentages of emergency room visits involving alcohol and

Table 7. Latino Drug-Related Emergency Room Visits, 2007

DRUG	# OF DRUG-RELATED VISITS	PERCENT*
Methamphetamines	25,483	18.6
Cocaine	49,810	36.4
Marijuana	49,593	36.2
Heroin	31,031	22.7
PCP	3,677	2.7
Ecstasy (MDMA)	3,089	2.3
Total	162,683	—

Source: Substance Abuse and Mental Health Services Administration, Drug Abuse Warning Network, 2011: National Estimates of Drug-Related Emergency Department Visits. HHS Publication No. (SMA) 13-4760, DAWN Series D-39. Rockville, MD: Substance Abuse and Mental Health Services Administration, 2013.

* Total percentages may exceed 100 percent due to multiple drug use during admission.

Table 8. Drug-Related Emergency Room Visits Involving Drugs and Alcohol Taken Together (as Percentage of All Admissions)

RACE/ETHNICITY	# OF ER VISITS	PERCENT
Non-Latino white	356,004	58.7
African American	135,296	22.3
Latino	66,174	10.9

Source: Substance Abuse and Mental Health Services Administration, Drug Abuse Warning Network, 2011: National Estimates of Drug-Related Emergency Department Visits. HHS Publication No. (SMA) 13-4760, DAWN Series D-39. Rockville, MD: Substance Abuse and Mental Health Services Administration, 2013.

illicit drugs. These emergency room admissions are further broken down into the percentage of drug users who had used a single drug versus a combination of drugs.

Drug-Related Deaths

DAWN defines a drug-related death as any death in which drug use is a contributory factor; drug use need not be the direct or sole cause of death. As a result some medical examiners may use circumstantial evidence in reporting drug-related deaths, whereas others may report only deaths confirmed through toxicological analysis. Thus, the information in table 9 should be viewed with these limitations in mind. According to the CDC, drug-induced deaths include all deaths for which drugs, excluding alcohol,

Table 9.   Drug-Induced Death Rates among Racial/Ethnic Groups, 2003–2007, United States

RACE/ETHNICITY	2003	2004	2005	2006	2007
Non-Latino white	8.0	8.9	9.6	10.8	11.4
Non-Latino black	6.6	6.8	7.4	7.9	7.5
Latino	3.3	3.4	3.5	3.9	3.4

Source: Leonard J. Paulozzi, "Drug-Induced Deaths: United States, 2003–2007," MMWR 60, no. 1 (January 14, 2011): 60–61.

are the underlying cause. As shown in table 9, Latinos have the lowest drug-induced death rates per 100,000 population.[39]

Other Adverse Health Effects of Substance Abuse

Beyond HIV/AIDS, drug overdoses, and drug-related deaths, there are several other adverse consequences of substance abuse. Particularly significant are the morbidity and mortality related to tobacco and alcohol consumption. Latinos, especially Mexican Americans, have higher prevalence rates of cirrhosis of the liver and chronic liver disease than do non-Latino whites. Additionally, the incidence of lung cancer and cardiovascular disease among Latinos is directly linked to the chronic use of tobacco products and alcohol. The use of alcohol and other drugs also contributes to unintentional injuries (such as motor vehicle accidents), which are the third leading cause of mortality among Latinos. Further, the use of alcohol, tobacco, and other drugs is associated with depression, antisocial personality, and organic brain damage. Needle sharing and lack of needle hygiene among IDUs lead to the increased prevalence and incidence of hepatitis B and hepatitis C.[40] Clearly, the association of substance use with other forms of morbidity and mortality will continue if steps are not taken to prevent substance use or to intervene with those who are presently using substances.

Prevention Issues among Latino Youth and Adolescents

> I recommend that today's young people . . . take education seriously so they would have less problems finding good jobs and a good place [healthy community] to live in. (Enrique A., 30)

We have seen that substance use among youth and adults involves a number of different and co-occurring factors. Taken together, these factors form the "web of causation" composed of individual characteristics, family characteristics, peer-group influences, and the general social environment. Despite the specific risk factors contributing to adolescent substance abuse, there are also resiliency and protective factors that can be marshaled to delay or prevent the initiation of substance use. These positive factors are not conceptualized as simply the opposite of risk factors. Rather, they interact with risk factors to mitigate, or lessen, their effect. The idea of identifying protective processes or specifying particular interactions among variables that produce resilience has direct relevance for risk-focused drug abuse prevention. Moreover, due to the interactive and often synergistic nature of many risk factors, prevention strategies should focus on simultaneously reducing multiple risks and enhancing multiple protective factors. Research has demonstrated that as protective factors increase, substance abuse decreases. Conversely, as risk factors increase, so does substance use.[41]

Four attributes have been consistently identified as describing resilient youth:

- *social competence*, which includes the qualities of responsiveness, flexibility, empathy, caring, communication skills, sense of humor, and pro-social behavior
- *problem solving*, which includes skills such as abstract, reflective, and flexible thinking and identifying multiple solutions for both cognitive and social problems
- *autonomy*, or a sense of one's own identity and the ability to act independently and exert some control over one's environment
- *a sense of purpose/future*, which includes healthy expectancies for the future, goal-directedness, success orientation, achievement motivation, educational aspirations, persistence, hopefulness, belief in a bright future, and a sense of coherence

Other factors critical to the positive development of youth are a caring, supportive family environment in which adults have high and clear expectations and provide children with opportunities to participate meaningfully in the family. Four general substance-abuse prevention strategies have been used with adolescents: providing knowledge and information, affective education (empathy and interpersonal skills), social-resistance skills training (for example, how to refuse drugs while maintaining friendships), and personal and social skills training.[42]

Approaches that provide information typically focus on the negative impact of substance use on academic performance, interpersonal relations, and social functioning. Additionally, these approaches provide information on patterns of drug use and the pharmacology of drugs. As Botvin notes, these approaches assume that given accurate information, people will make a rational decision about whether to use drugs.[43] In fact, however, information-based approaches have shown little effectiveness in changing behavior.

Effective education approaches emphasize the personal and social development of youth. Psychosocial factors in the etiology of substance use are a prime focus in this approach; for example, substance abuse tends to be correlated with low self-esteem and poor social skills. The theory is that intervening to improve social skills and self-esteem, without focusing directly on drugs, will make youth less vulnerable to substance use. Again, however, research studies have failed to demonstrate the effectiveness of this approach in reducing drug use.

Social resistance skills training appears to be a promising approach. This approach attempts to **psychologically inoculate** youth by giving them social skills to resist peer pressure to use drugs. Personal and social skills training emphasize the teaching of generic personal self-management skills and social skills. Examples include decision-making and problem-solving skills; cognitive skills for resisting peer, family, and media influences; skills for enhancing self-esteem; and adaptive coping responses, among others. This approach differs from the others in that it addresses a wide range of skills relevant to the youths' social environment. It appears to be a promising approach to reducing substance use among adolescents.

Interventions involving the families of Latino youth and adolescents have shown promising results in terms of reducing substance use and strengthening parent-child communication. A Brief Strategic Family Therapy intervention with Latino delinquent adolescents and their families was assessed by Santestiban and colleagues (2003) and found to be successful in reducing reports of delinquency and marijuana use among the adolescents involved.[44] More recent studies have shown positive effects of involving family in reducing substance use among Latino youth.[45]

Concluding Thoughts

The United States and other countries in Central and South America are undergoing dramatic social change in their attitudes about substance use, in particular the use of marijuana. Several countries, including Mexico, have decriminalized the use and possession of small amounts of marijuana (typically one ounce or less). In the United States the medical and recreational use of marijuana has been approved in several states (Arizona, California, Colorado, and Washington). What this portends for the health of the Latino population, especially youth and adolescents, remains to be seen.

Substance abuse continues to be a significant problem facing the Latino community. An individual's level of acculturation and nativity status is highly correlated with drug use: more acculturated Latinos and those born in the United States tend to have higher rates of use of legal and illegal substances than do less acculturated Latinos and those born in Mexico. More Mexican American males than females use legal and illegal drugs. Use of marijuana, inhalants, and heroin is greater among Mexican American adolescents than among non-Latino white adolescents. Injection drug users are a small but important group within the Latino population because Latinos are overrepresented in this segment of drug users.

Some studies have linked antisocial behavior to substance abuse, although it is unclear which comes first. The health consequences of drug use, however, are clear. For example, among Latino men, IDUs account for more than one-third of all reported AIDS cases; among Latina women, IDUs account for 41 percent of such cases. Within this subgroup, gay/bisexual IDUs pose an especially high risk to themselves as well as their sexual partners as a result of risky behavior associated with intravenous drug use. Mexican-origin women who are in a relationship with an IDU are also at risk for HIV even if they themselves are not IDUs. In addition, those women who are IDUs are just as likely to engage in risky drug-related and sexual behavior as non-Latina white women, thus increasing their exposure to HIV/AIDS. Other adverse health effects associated with substance abuse among Mexican Americans include hepatitis B and C, cirrhosis of the liver, chronic liver disease, lung cancer, cardiovascular disease, and high mortality and injury rates due to motor vehicle accidents.

Prevention of drug use as a means of reducing the risk for HIV/AIDS in the overall Latina population should focus on increasing awareness of the risks involved in taking drugs and having unprotected sex. Preventative measures include disseminating information, particularly in programs aimed at Latino youth, providing social-resistance skills training, and providing programs that are both culturally appropriate and culturally sensitive in their approaches to prevention strategies. Strategies may include providing information in Spanish, hiring bilingual/bicultural staff, aiming intervention at specific communities, recognizing cultural differences and values, and providing culturally sensitive health-care environments. Although providing intervention programs to reduce substance abuse and associated health risks is a challenge, there are established models that can be used in constructing a program that provides culturally competent and culturally sensitive interventions.[46]

Discussion Exercises

1. In what ways has HIV/AIDS affected the health status of the Mexican-origin population? What types of prevention options have been presented in this chapter?

2. How do the major HIV transmission categories differ among Latino subgroups and place of birth?

3. How does substance abuse among Mexican-origin persons differ from that among non-Latino whites, other Latino subpopulations, and African Americans?

4. What are the most common predictors of substance abuse among Mexican American adults and adolescents?

5. What types of drug-related behaviors pose the highest risks to the health status of the Mexican-origin community? How are Latino youth at risk?

6. Discuss the special health problems faced by Mexican-origin women.

7. How can cultural factors increase or decrease the risk for substance abuse? How can cultural concepts and beliefs be incorporated into substance-abuse prevention and intervention programs?

Notes

1. Many of the data in this section are for the Latino population because no data are available for the Mexican-origin subpopulation.

2. Centers for Disease Control and Prevention, "Diagnoses of HIV Infection and AIDS in the United States and Dependent Areas 2008," June 14–November 9, 2010, http://www.cdc.gov/.

3. Centers for Disease Control and Prevention, "Youth Risk Behavior Surveillance, United States, 2009," Surveillance Summaries, June 4, 2010. *Morbidity and Mortality Weekly Report* 59, no. SS-5 (2010).

4. L. D. Johnston, P. M. O'Malley, and J. G. Bachman, *The Monitoring the Future Study, 1975–1998*, vol. 1 (Washington, DC: National Institute on Drug Abuse, U.S. Department of Health and Human Services, National Institutes of Health, 1999).

5. National Institute on Drug Abuse (NIDA), *National Household Survey on Drug Abuse: Population Estimates 1991*, DHHS Pub. No. (ADM) 92–1887 (Washington, DC: U.S. Department of Health and Human Services, 1991).

6. P. D. Sorlie et al., "Design and Implementation of the Hispanic Community Health Study/Study of Latinos," *Annals of Epidemiology* 20, no.8 (August 2010): 629–41.

7. HHANES is the most important and comprehensive survey of Hispanic health. It focuses on areas with high concentrations of specific Hispanic subpopulations. The Mexican-origin persons surveyed for the HHANES were located in five southwestern states. See NIDA, *Use of Selected Drugs among Hispanics: Mexican-Americans, Puerto Ricans, and Cuban-Americans; Findings from the Hispanic Health and Nutrition Examination Survey* (Washington, DC: U.S. Department of Health and Human Services, Public Health Service, 1987).

8. *Results from the 2009 National Survey on Drug Use and Health: Volume I. Summary of National Findings*, NSDUH Series H-38A, HHS Publication No. SMA 10–4586 Findings (Rockville, MD: Substance Abuse and Mental Health Services Administration, Office of Applied Studies, 2010).

9. Substance Abuse and Mental Health Services Administration, *Prevalence of Substance Use among Racial & Ethnic Subgroups in the U.S., 1998*, retrieved on November 13, 2010, from http://oas.samhsa.gov/.

10. *The NSDUH Report: Injection Drug Use and Related Risk Behaviors* (Rockville, MD: Substance Abuse and Mental Health Services Administration, Office of Applied Studies, October 29, 2009), retrieved on November 13, 2010, from http://oas.samhsa.gov/.

11. NIDA, *National Household Survey on Drug Abuse*.

12. Ibid.

13. Impact Consultants, *School-Based Survey Report for 6th and 10th Graders in Yuma County, Arizona, 1995* (Tucson, AZ: Impact Consultants, 1995).

14. L. D. Johnston et al., *The Monitoring the Future Study* (Ann Arbor: University of Michigan, 2014).

15. Impact Consultants, *School-Based Survey Report for 6th and 10th Graders in Yuma County, Arizona, 1995* (Tucson, AZ: Impact Consultants, 1995).

16. *Drug Use among Racial/Ethnic Minorities*, NIH Publication No. 03–3888 (Bethesda, MD: National Institute on Drug Abuse, 2003).

17. Ibid.

18. M. Felix-Ortiz and M. D. Newcomb, "Cultural Identity and Drug Use among Latino and Latina Adolescents," in *Drug Abuse Prevention with Multiethnic Youth*, ed. G. J. Botvin, S. Schinke, and M. A. Orlandi, 147–68 (Thousand Oaks, CA: Sage, 1995).

19. Ibid., 150.

20. Borges et al., "A Cross-National Study on Mexico-US Migration, Substance Use and Substance Use Disorders," *Drug and Alcohol Dependence* 117 (2011): 16–23.

21. E. L. Chávez, R. Edwards, and E. R. Oetting, "Mexican American and White American Dropouts' Drug Use, Health Status, and Involvement in Violence," *Public Health Reports* 104, no. 6 (1986): 594–604.

22. Centers for Disease Control and Prevention, *HIV Surveillance Report, 2011*, vol. 23 (February 2013), retrieved on December 5, 2013, from http://www.cdc.gov/.

23. COSSMHO (National Coalition of Hispanic Health and Human Service Organizations), *HIV/AIDS—The Impact on Hispanics in Selected States* (Washington, DC: COSSMHO, 1991).

24. A. L. Estrada, "Drug Use and HIV Risks among African American, Mexican American, and Puerto Rican Drug Injectors," *Journal of Psychoactive Drugs* 30, no. 3 (1998): 247–53; see also I. D. Montoya, A. L. Estrada, A. Jones, and R. R. Robles, "An Analysis of Differential Factors Affecting Risk Behaviors among Out-of-Treatment Drug Users in Four Cities," *Drugs and Society* 9 (1996): 155–71; and R. R. Robles et al., "Effects of HIV Testing and Counseling on Reducing HIV Risk Behavior among Two Ethnic Groups," in *Multicultural AIDS Prevention Programs*, ed. R. Trotter (New York: Haworth Press, 1996).

25. A. L. Estrada, "Drug Use and HIV Risks among African American, Mexican American, and Puerto Rican Drug Injectors," *Journal of Psychoactive Drugs* 30, no. 3 (1998): 247–53. See also R. G. Deiss et al., "High-Risk Sexual and Drug Using Behaviors among Male Injection Drug Users Who Have Sex with Men in 2 Mexico-US Border Cities," *Sexually Transmitted Diseases* 35, no. 3 (March 2008): 243–49; K. C. Brouwer et al., "Estimated Numbers of Men and Women Infected with HIV/AIDS in Tijuana, Mexico," *Journal of Urban Health* 83 (2006): 299–307 [PubMed: 16736378]; T. L. Patterson et al., "Comparison of Sexual and Drug Use Behaviors between Female Sex Workers in Tijuana and Ciudad Juarez, Mexico," *Substance Use and Misuse* 41 (2006): 1535–49 [PubMed: 17002992]; C. Magis-Rodriguez et al., "HIV Prevalence and Correlates of Receptive Needle Sharing among Injection Drug Users in the Mexican-U.S. Border City of Tijuana," *Journal of Psychoactive Drugs* 37 (2005): 333–39 [PubMed: 16295018].

26. A. N. Martinez, R. N. Bluthenthal, N. M. Flynn, R. L. Anderson, and A. H. Kral, "HIV Risks and Seroprevalence among Mexican American Injection Drug Users in California," *AIDS Behavior*, Online First (2009).

27. R. E. Booth et al., "HIV Risk-Related Sex Behaviors among Injection Drug Users, Crack Smokers, and Injection Drug Users Who Smoke Crack," *American*

Journal of Public Health 83, no. 8 (1993): 1144–48; see also J. B. Cohen et al., "Women and IV Drugs: Parental and Heterosexual Transmission of Human Immunodeficiency Virus," *Journal of Drug Issues* 19, no. 1 (1989): 39–56; A. L. Estrada, "Behavioral Epidemiology of HIV Risks among Injection Drug Users: Comparative Assessment," paper presented to the HIV-AIDS Health Services Research and Delivery Conference, Agency for Health Care Policy and Research (AHCPR) Miami, FL, December 1991.

28. G. E. Ibañez, D. W. Purcell, R. Stall, J. T. Parsons, and C. A. Gómez, "Sexual Risk, Substance Abuse, and Psychological Distress in HIV-Positive Gay and Bisexual Men Who Also Inject Drugs," supplement, *AIDS* 19, no. S1 (2005): S49–S55.

29. A. Ritieni, J. Moskowitz, and M. Tholandi, "HIV/AIDS Misconceptions among Latinos: Findings from a Population-Based Survey," *Health Education & Behavior* 35, no. 2 (2006): 245–59.

30. The Henry J. Kaiser Family Foundation, *HIV/AIDS Policy Fact Sheet: The Global Impact of HIV/AIDS on Youth*, 2002, retrieved on November 17, 2010, from http://www.pbs.org/.

31. S. M. Kegeles et al., "Sexually Active Adolescents and Condoms: Changes over One Year in Knowledge, Attitudes, and Use," *American Journal of Public Health* 78 (1988): 460–61.

32. E. Norris and K. Ford, "Condom Beliefs in Urban, Low Income, African American and Hispanic Youth," *Health Education and Behavior* 21, no. 1 (1994): 39–53.

33. D. S. Moore and P. I. Erickson, "Age, Gender, and Ethnic Differences in Sexual and Contraceptive Knowledge, Attitudes, and Behaviors," *Family and Community Health* 8 (1985): 38–51.

34. D. C. Des Jarlais et al., "Heterosexual Partners: A Large Risk Group for AIDS" [letter], *Lancet* 2, no. 8415 (1984): 1346–47.

35. J. Mondanaro, *Treating Chemically Dependent Women* (Lexington, MA: Lexington Books, 1988).

36. G. Weissman et al., "Drug Use and Sexual Behaviors among Sex Partners of Injecting-Drug Users, United States, 1988–1990," *Mortality and Morbidity Weekly Report* 40, no. 49 (1991): 855–60.

37. S. J. Stevens, J. R. Erickson, and A. L. Estrada, "Characteristics of Female Sexual Partners of Injection Drug Users in Southern Arizona: Implications for Effective HIV Risk Reduction Interventions," *Drugs and Society* 7, no. 3/4 (1993): 129–42.

38. *Drug Abuse Warning Network, 2007: National Estimates of Drug-Related Emergency Department Visits* (Rockville, MD: Substance Abuse and Mental Health Services Administration, Office of Applied Studies, 2010), retrieved from http://www.samhsa .gov/.

39. L. V. Paulozzi, "Drug Induced Deaths—United States, 2003–2007," *Morbidity and Mortality Weekly Report* 60, no. 1 (January 14, 2011): 60–61, retrieved on July 12, 2011, from http://www.cdc.gov/.

40. A. L. Estrada, "Health Disparities among African American and Hispanic Drug Injectors: HIV, AIDS, Hepatitis B Virus, Hepatitis C Virus: A Review," supplement, *AIDS* 19, no. S3 (2005): S4–S52.

41. Felix-Ortiz and Newcomb, "Cultural Identity and Drug Use among Latino and Latina Adolescents," in *Drug Abuse Prevention with Multiethnic Youth*, ed. G. J. Botvin, S. Schinke, and M. A. Orlandi, 147–68. (Thousand Oaks, CA: Sage, 1995).

42. G. J. Botvin, "Drug Abuse Prevention in School Settings," in *Drug Abuse Prevention with Multiethnic Youth*, ed. G. J. Botvin, S. Schinke, and M. A. Orlandi, 169–92 (Thousand Oaks, CA: Sage, 1995).

43. Ibid.

44. D. A. Santisteban et al., "Efficacy of Brief Strategic Family Therapy in Modifying Hispanic Adolescent Behavior Problems and Substance Use," *Journal of Family Psychology* 17, no. 1 (2003): 121–33.

45. L. R. Williams, S. L. Ayers, M. M. Garvey, "Efficacy of a Culturally Based Parenting Intervention: Strengthening Open Communication Between Mexican-Heritage Parents and Adolescent Children," *Journal of the Society for Social Work and Research* 3, no. 4 (December 3, 2012): 296–307.

46. HIV/AIDS Prevention Research Synthesis Project, retrieved on July 11, 2011, from http://www.CDC.gov/.

Suggested Readings

Akins, C., and G. Beschner. *Ethnography: A Research Tool for Policy Makers in the Drug and Alcohol Fields.* Rockville, MD: NIDA, 1980.

Botvin, G. J. "Drug Abuse Prevention in School Settings." In *Drug Abuse Prevention with Multiethnic Youth*, ed. G. J. Botvin, S. Schinke, and M. A. Orlandi, 169–92. Thousand Oaks, CA: Sage, 1995.

Bullington, B. M. *Heroin in the Barrio.* Lexington, MA: Lexington Press, 1977.

Felix-Ortiz, M., and M. D. Newcomb. "Cultural Identity and Drug Use among Latino and Latina Adolescents." In *Drug Abuse Prevention with Multiethnic Youth*, ed. G. J. Botvin, S. Schinke, and M. A. Orlandi, 147–68. Thousand Oaks, CA: Sage, 1995.

Glick, R., and J. Moore, eds. *Drug Use in Hispanic Communities.* New Brunswick, NJ: Rutgers University Press, 1990.

Hanson, B. *Life with Heroin: Voices from the Inner City.* Lexington, MA: Lexington Books, 1985.

Mondanaro, J. *Treating Chemically Dependent Women.* Lexington, MA: Lexington Books, 1988.

Moore, J. W., and R. Garcia. *Homeboys: Gangs, Drugs and Prison in the Barrios of Los Angeles.* Philadelphia: Temple University Press, 1978.

Padilla, F. *The Gang as an American Enterprise.* Brunswick, NJ: Rutgers University Press, 1992.

Robles, R. R., T. D. Matos, H. M. Colon, C. A. Marrero, and J. C. Reyes. "Effects of HIV Testing and Counseling on Reducing HIV Risk Behavior among Two Ethnic Groups." In *Multicultural AIDS Prevention Programs*, ed. R. Trotter. New York: Haworth Press, 1996.

Rogler, L. H., R. G. Malgady, G. Costantino, and R. Blumenthal. "What Do Culturally Sensitive Mental Health Services Mean? The Case of Hispanics." *American Psychologist* 42 (1987): 565–70.

Santisteban, D., and J. Szapocnik. *The Hispanic Substance Abuser: The Search for Prevention Strategies.* New York: Grune and Stratton, 1982.

Singer, M., Z. Jia, J. J. Schensul, M. Weeks, and J. B. Page. "AIDS and the IV Drug User: The Local Context in Prevention Efforts." In *Rethinking AIDS Prevention: Cultural Approaches*, ed. R. Bolton and M. Singer, 147–68. New York: Gordon and Breach Science Publishers, 1992.

Chapter 4

Health-Care Access

"Treated Like Second-Class Citizens"

There was no medical insurance in my family. . . . Grandma would pay. At that time we had doctors that did home visits. As a matter of fact, I remember having an asthma attack and the doctor coming to visit me. (María L., 44)

I initially told [the doctor] that I was on [the Arizona Health Care Cost Containment System] AHCCCS[1] because of the circumstance, not by choice, that I was a professional and that I was used to having my own medical insurance, because somehow I felt that I would be treated differently [than a non-AHCCCS patient] . . . and I feel that I was right. . . . The impression I had about AHCCCS patients . . . is that they are [treated like] second-class citizens. (Carmen G., 49)

Like many Mexican Americans, both María and Carmen experienced the dilemma of not having health insurance or the security of private health insurance coverage. As a child growing up in San Diego, California, María did not have health insurance and therefore had to rely on her grandmother to pay for the family's health care. Carmen's case illustrates the problem of losing health insurance due to unforeseen circumstances. She was forced to give up her job, resulting in the loss of her private health coverage, and move from Colorado back to Arizona to care for her ailing mother. These two women clearly illustrate the dilemmas of financial access to health care, that is, having either private or public health insurance to pay for medical services. This problem is widespread and often linked to employment factors such as occupational location (including economic sector and business size), part-time versus full-time status, salary, and immigration status. The passage of the PPACA, more commonly known as Obamacare, in 2010 may change some of the disparities in care due to financial access. Before examining the specific coverage problems faced by the Mexican-origin population, we must define health-care access.

What Is Health-Care Access?

Indicators of access to health care include having a regular source of care, having health insurance coverage, and the rates at which barriers prevented access to health care. One of the more enduring frameworks for assessing access to health care was proposed by Andersen and colleagues and more recently expanded by Gelberg, Andersen, and Leake (2000) and Stein, Andersen, and Gelberg (2007).[2] This model was developed to predict health-care utilization among "vulnerable populations" such as racial/ ethnic groups, the homeless, the elderly, and the undocumented. The model consists of three main categories of predictors: predisposing predictors (e.g., demographic and social structure variables), enabling predictors (e.g., having a regular source of care, insurance coverage, and other personal and family resources), and health status predictors (e.g., health conditions, perceived health), all of which predict health behavior (e.g., personal health practices) and health outcomes (e.g., health status, satisfaction with care, realized access).

The issue of health-care access is significant to the health status of all Mexican Americans. Aspects that specifically affect this population include financial access to care, geographic access to care, access to timely care, having a regular source of care, access to culturally and linguistically appropriate care, and access to specialized types of health care. In many respects, we can divide access issues for the Mexican-origin population into two broad categories: (1) financial access and eligibility to care and (2) access to culturally and linguistically competent health-care professionals that serve predominately Mexican-origin communities. The latter point also encompasses the issues of location of delivery and timely and appropriate care. As we will see later in this chapter, access to a regular source of care for minority populations is linked to the availability of minority and/or culturally and linguistically competent health professionals in local areas.

Health-care access is important because it influences health status and quality of life. According to Williams and Torrens, "Poor access may be reflected in delayed care seeking, absence of preventive care, and low patient satisfaction."[3] These problems are illustrated by Carmen's loss of private health insurance, which affected not only her health but also the quality of health care she received:

Prior to the last six months I did have medical insurance available to me because, of course, I was working. I would definitely say that since January of this year, not having had medical insurance until May definitely affected my health because my body became weaker and weaker.... It's such a shame because medicine is supposed to be all about healing and helping and it's turned into such a money monopoly. (Carmen G., 49)

Unfortunately, Carmen's sentiments and experiences are all too familiar to Mexican Americans. For this population, the lack of health-care coverage and access is a barrier that prevents many from having a regular source of care that provides routine checkups and timely treatment of illnesses and diseases. Another concern is the shortage of health-care professionals who are knowledgeable in managing treatment for Latinos. As we will discover later in this chapter, the shortage of Latino, particularly Mexican American, health-care professionals limits access to care for this group. The cost of care also increases as Mexican-origin persons who are denied access to regular care must seek treatment in hospital emergency rooms when an illness has become unmanageable or life-threatening. These costs are paid by the state in the case of public health insurance and by the individual in the case of private insurance or no insurance.[4] This problem is often exacerbated by the use of alternative forms of treatment either prior to or in place of consulting a physician. For example, in the border region, Mexican-origin persons may receive health care in neighboring Mexican states, which lowers their out-of-pocket expenses or enables them to self-medicate by using pharmaceuticals that do not require a prescription.

Who Are the Uninsured?

Before the passage and implementation of the PPACA more than forty-five million Americans were without any form of health insurance; slightly more than six million of these uninsured were children under eighteen years of age.[5] Although more non-Latino whites were uninsured, the Latino population had a disproportionate percentage of uninsured: Latinos constituted roughly 16 percent of the U.S. population, yet they made up 32 percent of the uninsured population. In contrast, non-Latino whites represented 65 percent of the U.S. population but made up only 46 percent of Americans with no health insurance.[6] Between 1990 and 2000 the number of uninsured Latinos increased by 60 percent, from 7 million to 11.2 million. Another way to examine the same data is to track the percentage of uninsured within each ethnic and racial group. Within the three major ethnic and racial categories, Latinos are disproportionately uninsured: More than one-third of all Latinos do not have any form of health insurance, compared to less than one-fifth of all African Americans and one-tenth of all non-Latino whites.[7] With the introduction of the PPACA, as many as 95 percent of American citizens will receive healthcare coverage by the time the Act is fully implemented.

Financial Access to Care: A Crisis for Mexican-Origin Patients

> I was sick one time for five years because I had blood coming out of my mouth. For a lot of years I didn't know why it was coming out. I used to have a health plan maybe ten years ago. . . . I had a sore throat for two years, and it wasn't until I went to a county facility that the doctor explained to me that I had acid reflux. (Danny F., 36)

The issue of financial access to adequate health insurance is the major focus of discussion within the domain of health care coverage for many Latinos, particularly the Mexican-origin population. Before the PPACA, the inability to pay was the most significant barrier to a regular source of health care for this group; with the passage of PPACA, immigration status may become the most significant barrier to health care. The estimated eleven million undocumented immigrants residing in the United States, who are typically young, in the workforce, and in good health, will be excluded from participation in the new insurance marketplaces and Medicaid expansions by the states. Because uninsured individuals must pay for the cost of care out-of-pocket, they underutilize preventative services and delay treatment for both chronic and life-threatening conditions. Danny's case shows the impact of a lack of financial access to health care over a long period of time. The problem he was diagnosed with, acid reflux disease, is an easily treated gastrointestinal problem. Early diagnosis and treatment would have improved his quality of life and prevented his costly use of patchwork providers (those who treat the underinsured or uninsured), a method the uninsured and underinsured in California commonly use to treat various medical conditions. While

Danny's experience is not unique, it illustrates the problems resulting from a health-care financing and delivery system that is based on the employment status of the individual.

Private Health Insurance: An Employer-Based Model

As the cost of health care, particularly for care resulting from catastrophic illnesses, exceeds the price that most Americans are able to pay, health insurance becomes vital in ensuring quality of life and the continuity of health-care services. Without private or public health insurance, individuals may be denied treatment or services except in medical emergencies, which can result in long-term damage to their health.

Most Americans obtain access to health insurance through the workplace; as much as 55 percent of individuals are covered through Employer-Based Private Insurance (EBPI). Employers, particularly large firms and the public sector (including the government), typically provide health insurance to an individual and his or her family members as part of a comprehensive benefits package. This type of coverage is known as a **voluntary system of health insurance**. An individual employee either shares the **health insurance premium** with the employer or is provided with coverage at no cost. This coverage usually extends to the employee's family for a relatively small increase in cost, which is usually paid through regular premiums. In general, access to private health insurance is linked to the type, site, and duration of employment. These factors significantly influence the profile of uninsured Americans. For example, companies that provide full-coverage health insurance tend to be large private and public employers. Even within large companies, lower-paid employees or part-time workers may not receive healthcare benefits. The private sector includes corporations and businesses; the public sector includes school districts, universities, and governmental (or quasi-governmental) entities. EBPI provides coverage for families, but historically women and minorities have been left out of the system. Employers that do not typically provide health insurance to their employees include small businesses in competitive markets, such as landscaping, and those who employ persons such as domestic workers or child-care providers. Self-employed professionals such as lawyers, accountants, independent contractors, and consultants may also not have access to affordable health coverage. This type of employment frequently limits access to private insurance, as small employers often cannot afford to pay the health insurance premium to cover the cost of an employee's health insurance. The PPACA will try to rectify this issue by providing subsidies to small businesses to help them provide health care for their employees.

The Public Sector: Limited Access to Public-Sector Health Insurance

> The hours I work do not qualify me for part-time status to get part-time benefits, so therefore I didn't qualify to receive health insurance.... In February of this year, I twisted my knee and I was barely able to walk on it, but was hesitant to have anybody look at it because of the cost of not having any insurance.... Had I gone to the hospital and had X-rays taken and everything else, then I would have this thousand-dollar, if not more, medical bill that I could not pay for. So that's why not having health insurance has prevented me from seeking medical attention. (Marissia Q., 22)

The Personal Responsibility and Work Opportunity Act passed by Congress and signed by President Clinton in 1996 brought significant changes in publicly subsidized services for the poor and **medically indigent**. Yet, even before these changes, the Mexican-origin population in the United States did not use public health insurance programs as much as other racial and ethnic groups did. This may be due in part to the fact that a significant percentage of the Mexican-origin population is composed of recent immigrants, whose status affects their eligibility for federally subsidized health care. Today, even with the PPACA health care insurance reforms, undocumented immigrants cannot receive health-care subsidies. In addition, in many states, efforts to enroll this population are limited due to the limited resources available at local levels to promote outreach programs in a culturally sensitive manner. This inability, in turn, creates barriers due to the unfamiliarity of the Mexican-origin population with the availability and eligibility requirements of these programs. Moreover, in many of the states where the majority of the Mexican-origin population resides, there are stringent income eligibility

Table 10. Medicaid Coverage by Population Group, 2009

	NONCITIZENS (%)	NATURALIZED CITIZENS (%)	NATIVE-BORN (%)
Black	4.2	1.9	93.9
Latino	15.2	6.2	78.6
Asian	27.6	27.3	45.0
White	2.2	2.2	95.6

Source: U.S. Census Bureau, *Current Population Survey, Annual Social and Economic (ASEC) Supplement, 2009* (Washington, DC: Government Printing Office, 2010).

requirements in addition to county or state requirements that limit access to these public programs. Thus, factors such as low income, citizenship status, regional differences in awareness and eligibility requirements for publicly subsidized programs, and limited outreach to eligible individuals within this ethnic group combine to produce low enrollment rates for Mexican-origin persons in public programs that provide financial coverage for health-care services.

The impact of immigrant status on the use of publicly subsidized health insurance is illustrated in table 10. In 2009, native-born Latinos had a higher use of Medicaid than naturalized and non-citizen Latinos. The percentage of native-born Latinos receiving Medicaid is almost four times that of noncitizen and naturalized Latino immigrants. However, although Asian native-born immigrants have lower Medicaid utilization than Latino native-born individuals, they have a significantly higher use of Medicaid in their naturalized and noncitizen population relative to Latinos, which suggests that their immigrant status may not have the same degree of adverse impact. Given that Latinos are the largest immigrant group in the United States and that the Mexican-origin population is the largest subpopulation within this group, these data highlight the nuanced impact of immigration status on Medicaid utilization within the Latino population and across other immigrant groups.

Medicaid, Medicare, SCHIP, and SSI:
A Brief Overview

Four major federal health-care programs target people who are medically at-risk, disabled, children, or elderly. These are Medicaid, **Supplemental**

Security Income (SSI), Medicare, and **State Children's Health Insurance Program** (SCHIP). SSI is "a nationwide federal assistance program administered by the Social Security Administration (SSA) that guarantees a minimum level of income for needy aged, blind, or disabled individuals."[8]

Given the youthful character and relatively large family size of Mexican Americans, Medicaid and SCHIP eligibility criteria are of great interest in the examination of the group's overall health-care access. According to the Encyclopedia of Business:

> As the nation's second-largest health insurance program, Medicaid provides medical assistance to 36 million low-income Americans. It was established through Title XIX of the Social Security Act of 1965 to pay the health-care costs for members of society who otherwise could not afford treatment. The program is jointly funded by the federal government and the state governments, but is administered separately by each state within broad federal guidelines. Medicaid recipients include adults, children, and families, as well as elderly, blind, and disabled persons, who have low or no income and receive other forms of public assistance. Medicaid also covers the 'medically needy,' or those whose income is significantly reduced by large medical expenses.[9]

The groups covered under Medicaid include pregnant women, children, the elderly, and the disabled.

However, Medicaid did not provide enough benefits for the working poor, so SCHIP was created in 1997 to fill in the cracks for children of low-income families. States manage their own SCHIPs and can provide outreach and broader eligibility requirements in order to cover more children. While SCHIP seemed like a promising reform to provide coverage to low-income children who did not qualify for Medicaid, fluctuating eligibility requirements in the late 1990s and early 2000s posed barriers to enrollment. However, as the 2000s progressed, there was an increasing trend toward making programs like SCHIP more accessible. Additionally, the government increased funds for public insurance for children, from $18 million in 1987 to $30 million in 2007.

Although this working definition applies to the general application of these programs, each state has discretion in determining eligibility. However, there are requirements that states must meet in order to obtain eligible Medicaid and SCHIP funds from the federal government. For example, as mentioned previously, states must provide Medicaid coverage to individuals "who have low or no income and receive other forms of public assistance."[10]

States also have some discretion in determining the level of coverage based on their willingness to subsidize the health insurance program targeted to the poor and medically indigent. This has resulted in regional differences that may partially explain why the Mexican-origin population has differential access to publicly subsidized health insurance. Table 11 lists the selected Medicaid eligibility requirements for adults in the five southwestern states. It provides a good example of the diversity of state requirements for the Medicaid population.

Table 11. Selected Medicaid Eligibility Requirements for Adults in Five Southwestern States

STATE	INCOME REQUIREMENT	ADDITIONAL REQUIREMENTS
Arizona (AHCCCS/SOBRA)	133% of FPL* or less	Social Security number, state resident, U.S. citizen or qualified immigrant
California (Medi-Cal)	133% of FPL or less	Largely eligible with a few exceptions
Colorado (BCKC adult)	133% of FPL or less	State resident, U.S. citizen or qualified immigrant
New Mexico	133% of FPL or less	U.S. citizen or qualified immigrant
Texas	15% of FPL or less for adult parents and 9% for other adults	Social Security number, state resident, U.S. citizen or qualified immigrant, opted out Medicaid expansion

Source: Arizona Health Care Cost Containment System website: http://www.azahcccs .gov/; California Department of Health Care Services website:http://www.dhcs.ca.gov/; Colorado Consumer Health Initiative: "Connecting Care and Health in Colorado: A Guide To Services For The Uninsured" at http://cohealthinitiative.org/; "Medicaid Eligibility Manual," *New Mexico Human Services Register* 37, no. 12 (February, 2014), website: http:// www.hsd.state.nm.us/; "State Medicaid and CHIP Income Eligibility Standards," in Centers for Medicare and Medicaid Services, Center for Medicaid and Chip services website: http:// www.medicaid.gov/.
* The Federal Poverty Line (FPL) is the guideline for determining poverty status in the United States. The yearly income limit for a family of four to be in poverty is $23,850 in the lower forty-eight states and the District of Columbia.

In addition, the importance of proving legal status varies by state, thus affecting access for the undocumented immigrant population for public programs or the health insurance marketplace set up by PPACA. The more generous eligibility requirements and coverage in states such as California should provide Latinos with greater access. However, even with more generous coverage based on a higher poverty threshold, the citizenship status of undocumented immigrants influences the accessibility of publicly subsidized health insurance for the poor members of this subpopulation. Thus, even in states with relatively generous eligibility requirements, the relation of citizenship status to health-care access has become a serious issue as most state and federal benefits are either linked to duration of legal status or limited by the lack of proof of legal entry into the United States.

Medicare is a federal public health insurance program that was created primarily for the elderly. It covers people who are sixty-five years or older, individuals with permanent kidney failure, and people with certain disabilities. Unlike Medicaid, there is no income or eligibility means test for this program. Entitlement is based on employee payment into the Medicare trust. To qualify for Medicare, either the individual or his or her spouse must work for a minimum of ten years in a Medicare-covered job and be a permanent resident or citizen.[11] In some respects, Medicare may be viewed as a universal insurance program for America's senior citizens. There are two parts to the Medicare program. Medicare Part A, which covers most of the U.S. population aged sixty-five and older, is known as hospital insurance and provides the following benefits: ninety days of **inpatient care**, sixty reserve inpatient days for individuals who exhaust their ninety days, one hundred days of care in a skilled nursing facility after leaving the hospital, and **home health agency** visits. Part B of the Medicare program is a supplemental health insurance program paid for through monthly premiums. It covers preventative screenings, physician services, **outpatient health services**, and home health care for those not covered by Part A.[12]

Table 12 compares Medicare and Medicaid before and after the implementation of the PPACA. The PPACA will increase the number of individuals and the types of coverage provided by these two federal programs. Individuals at a lower income level will be covered by Medicaid, and items like prescription drugs will be more fully covered under Medicare.

Table 12. Comparison of Coverage under Medicaid, Medicare, and PPACA

	BEFORE PPACA		AFTER PPACA	
	MEDICAID	MEDICARE	MEDICAID	MEDICARE
People covered	Low income and disabled	People over age 65 and disabled	Low income and disabled	People over age 65 and disabled
Coverage changes	Less community-based coverage, less in-home care for people with disabilities	Had to pay for preventative services, prescription drug "donut hole"	Increased community-based coverage, more in-home care for people with disabilities	Reduced prescription drug costs, increased preventative services, one free wellness checkup per year
Cost	Cost sharing depends on state, designed to be low to make coverage affordable	Some cost sharing of services with the program	To cover more individuals, federal government will fully fund Medicaid until 2020	More services fully covered, reducing the cost sharing required

Sources: HealthCare.gov, "Qualifying for Medicaid coverage" website: http://www.health care.gov/; HealthCare.gov, "Medicare & the Marketplace" website: http://www.healthcare .gov/; Medicaid.gov, "Affordable Care Act" website: http://www.medicaid.gov/.

The Patient Protection and Affordable Care Act

The PPACA of 2010, more commonly known as Obamacare, has become the most significant and controversial reform of the health-care system since the establishment of Medicare and Medicaid in 1965 and will drastically change healthcare policy in the United States. Previous to its passage, individuals received health insurance either through an employer (55.1 percent), through the purchase of direct private insurance (9.8 percent), or through a government program such as Medicare (32.2 percent). This left 15.7 percent of individuals in the United States uninsured. Within the U.S. Latino population, however, 30.1 percent were uninsured. With the introduction of the PPACA, a projected 95 percent of American citizens will receive healthcare coverage beginning in 2014, when the Act completes its first stage of implementation. However, a recent report by the Department of Health and Human Services indicates that this enrollment goal may not be met. Only eight million Americans had enrolled in a Marketplace plan as of April 2014. Of these, 28 percent were between the ages of eighteen and thirty-four.[13] In California, only 22 percent of eligible Latinos had enrolled as of early 2014. The enrollment of Latinos is critical given their relatively younger age and better health status, which would help keep the PPACA premiums low. The comprehensive law includes stronger consumer rights and protections, more affordable coverage, better access to health care, and modifications to contain Medicare costs. The law, however, precludes benefits for undocumented immigrant families.

The PPACA is designed based on a three-point formula that seeks to increase the number of individuals who have access to health-care insurance. These three points include the establishment of stronger consumer rights and protections that limit the ability of insurance companies to decline individual applications due to preexistent conditions. The law also creates incentives for individuals, employers, and insurance companies to participate in the program. For example, to minimize insurance companies' risk of adverse selection as a result of enrolling a disproportionate share of less healthy members, the Act requires mandatory health-care insurance for all individuals. To positively induce all consumers to enroll in an insurance program, the PPACA provides subsidies for those individuals who need financial assistance. Finally, the PPACA introduced a series of Patient's Rights that seek to empower individuals in their selection and use of health care.

Table 13 compares the difference in coverage between EBPI before the implementation of the PPACA and EBPI after the PPACA. The PPACA expands coverage in almost all areas and requires all providers of health insurance policies to follow these new guidelines. The only exceptions are plans that are "grandfathered" in or plans bought before the PPACA went into effect.

Figure 19 shows the hypothetical subsidies that a family of four would receive for the Covered California health insurance exchange. The amount of subsidies a household receives is based on the number of individuals living in the household, separated by children and adults, and the income of the household. Families have different options for the amount of coverage they receive through the exchange, and families can choose to pay more out of pocket for a higher benefits plan.

Even though some progress has been made over the past century toward the creation of a national health-care system, drastic policy changes still need to be made if health disparities due to income level and place of employment are to be eliminated. Popular opinion in the late 2000s was in favor of system-wide health-care reform, but the general public was wary

Table 13. Difference in Coverage between EBPI before PPACA and EBPI after PPACA

	EBPI BEFORE PPACA	EBPI AFTER PPACA
Preexisting conditions (adults)	Coverage could be limited or denied	May be covered under PCIP until 2014, after 2014 guaranteed coverage
Preexisting conditions (children)	Coverage could be limited or denied	Guaranteed coverage
Age of children under parent's plan	Usually age 19 (maybe later if full-time student)	Required coverage through age 26
Limits on lifetime/annual coverage	Set by insurance company, patients pay anything over that amount	No limits allowed on "Essential Health Benefits"
Primary care physician	May be chosen by insurance company; OB-GYN may require a referral	Patient chooses any primary care provider in the insurance network; no referral for OB-GYN
Emergency care outside of network	Insurance companies may charge for out-of-network care	Guaranteed coverage
Premium dollars spent	May be spent on administrative costs	80% of premium dollars must be spent on health-care costs
Coverage withdrawal	Insurance companies can withdraw coverage if a mistake is made on insurance application	Insurance companies cannot withdraw coverage because of an honest mistake
Increases in coverage	Insurance companies can increase rates at their discretion	Unreasonable cost increases must be publicly stated and justified

Source: HealthCare.gov, "Health coverage rights and protections" website: https://www
.healthcare.gov/.
Notes: EBPI: Employer-based private insurance; PPACA: Patient Protection and Affordable
Care Act; PCIP: Preexisting Condition Insurance Plan; "Essential Health Benefits" outlined
by PPACA.

of increased government spending, especially in light of the Great Recession in 2008. People were reluctant to pay more taxes to support health-care reform when their household finances were not stable. Historically, Americans have been against tax increases and have voted against programs that would increase taxes.

A family of four: Marta, 36, David, 35, Marisol, 10, and Juan, 8, live in California. Marta and David were both born in Mexico but are now legal residents of the United States. Under the Affordable Care Act, Marta and David have to purchase health insurance for their family. Marta and David do not receive health insurance coverage through their employers, so they decide to purchase insurance through the California Health Benefits Exchange, also called Covered California. Together, Marta and David earn $45,000 per year, which makes them over-qualified for Medi-Cal, California's Medicaid program. Through the Health Benefits Exchange, based on their income, their ages, and the ages of Marisol and Juan, Marta and David can expect to pay roughly $1,034 per month in insurance. However, Marta and David can receive $750 per month in tax credits from the government to help them receive affordable insurance. With the credits, Marta and David will have to pay $284 per month for their insurance coverage.

Source: IRS, "Health Coverage Tax Credit: Eligibility Requirements and How to Receive the Health Coverage Tax Credit": http://www.irs.gov/.

Figure 19. California hypothetical subsidies.

The 2012 presidential election became an important battleground for health-care reform.[14] Parts of the PPACA had already gone into effect, and millions of dollars had been invested in national health care. If President Obama had not been reelected, not only would the law likely have been repealed but the money that had already gone toward its implementation would have been wasted. On November 6, 2012, Barack Obama was reelected, and the future of the PPACA seemed relatively secure under his administration. However, strong political opposition to the implementation of the PPACA by key Republican congressional leaders and governors created viable threats to the successful implementation of this important health-care reform law.

While the PPACA will likely improve the overall health-care insurance coverage for Mexican Americans, there are pending aspects of Mexican American health care that the Act does not address. These factors, such as culturally and linguistically sensitive care, may still limit the quality of care that Mexican Americans receive.

Risk Factors that Influence the Health Insurance Coverage of the Mexican-Origin Population

Much of the Mexican-origin population falls within the category of the working poor. This means that while they are employed in low-wage employment sectors that do not provide health insurance, their incomes do

Table 14. Percentage of Population under Age Sixty-Five Having Private Insurance Coverage Obtained through the Workplace, 2005–2007

RACE/ETHNICITY	2005	2006	2007
White, non-Latino	71.9	69.9	70.2
Black, non-Latino	50.9	49.5	49.5
Asian	64.4	64.5	64.6
All Latino	40.0	37.7	38.8
Mexican	37.6	34.9	35.7

Source: National Center for Health Statistics, Health, United States, 2009, table 138 (Hyattsville, MD: U.S. Department of Health and Human Services, 2010).

not meet the federal poverty levels required for publicly subsidized health insurance. The PPACA will try to help the working poor by providing subsidies to help families and individuals pay for insurance. Compounding this problem, the Mexican-origin population aged sixty-five and older has a very low rate of private health insurance coverage provided through previous employment, leaving them entirely dependent on Medicare.[15]

Occupational Location

Occupational location refers to the type of job and economic sector in which a person is employed. At the low end of the spectrum are low-status, low-wage jobs such as those in the agricultural and service sectors, while at the high end are corporate executives, doctors, lawyers, and other white-collar jobs. Compared to black and white non-Latinos, Asians, and other Latinos, the Mexican-origin population under the age of sixty-five had the lowest rate of private insurance obtained through employment (see table 14). Given the low occupational status of a large percentage of the Mexican-origin population of the United States, particularly in the Southwest, it is not surprising that private health insurance coverage among this population is relatively low.

Eligibility Issues for Latino Seniors

As illustrated in table 15, the Latino population aged sixty-five and older has a very low rate of private health insurance coverage provided through previous employment programs, compared to white and black non-Latinos. The significance of this situation is that, unlike the 37 percent of non-Latino whites who have private health insurance to complement or replace their Medicare coverage, most of the senior Latino population must rely

Table 15. Percentage of Population Age Sixty-Five and Older Having Private Insurance Coverage Obtained through the Workplace, 2000, 2006, 2007

RACE/ETHNICITY	2000	2006	2007
White, non-Latino	38.6	37.1	36.8
Black, non-Latino	22.0	23.7	25.8
Latino	15.8	17.1	16.2

Source: National Center for Health Statistics, Health, United States, 2009, table 141 (Hyattsville, MD: U.S. Department of Health and Human Services, 2010).

on Medicare to cover the bulk of their health-care costs. This also reflects their occupational location in low-wage and low-benefit sectors of the economy during their prime working years. Before the PPACA, this group of seniors generally had no coverage for prescription drugs and other medical expenses not covered under Medicare. Lack of supplemental insurance places an enormous financial burden on these low-income seniors, who have fixed incomes from Social Security or private pension plans. Because of the substantial out-of-pocket expenses, many do not follow through with regular treatment or medications for common chronic conditions such as diabetes, high blood pressure, or heart disease. According to the most recent data released from the Department of Health and Human Services, few seniors have enrolled in PPACA.

Mexican-Origin Women: A Group at Risk

[The lack of access] is reflected in very low levels of utilization of screening technologies among women (e.g. **Pap smear**, mammography, etc.). . . . An understanding of the epidemiology and biology of many disease processes (e.g., cervical cancer and HPV disease) in high-risk populations would greatly advance our understanding of these illnesses. (Francisco G., MD, 35)

A significant number of Mexican-origin women either are not able to work full time because of family obligations or are employed in low-wage sectors. As a result they do not have access to health insurance. This is illustrated in table 16, which shows the percentage of Mexican-origin women who have private health insurance or Medicaid.

With the exception of those aged sixty-five and older, approximately one-third of Mexican-origin women do not have any source of payment for their health care. These data become even more alarming when we

Table 16. Percentage of Mexican-Origin Women Having Private or Public Health Insurance Coverage (n = 10,231)

AGE RANGE (YEARS)	PERCENTAGE
25–44	57.2
45–54	66.9
55–64	65.9
≥ 65	93.7

Source: J. L. Angel, J. K. Montez, and R. J. Angel, "A Window of Vulnerability: Health Insurance Coverage Among Women 55 to 64 Years of Age," *Women's Health Issues* (2010). Available online at http://www.whijournal.com/.

review women who are no longer in their childbearing years but are not old enough to qualify for Medicare. Many chronic health conditions, such as diabetes and cardiovascular disease, manifest themselves after age forty, but women in this age bracket who lack health insurance cannot receive timely screening and monitoring of these diseases to minimize their adverse health effects. Moreover, older uninsured women are at greater risk of remaining undiagnosed and untreated for life-threatening diseases such as breast cancer and cervical cancer, which have few early symptoms. Preventative screenings and care is very important for detecting diseases that more often affect women. Thus, the poor health status of these women can be directly linked to their lack of financial access to health insurance.[16] The PPACA tries to help solve this problem by providing subsidies and preventative care to women without insurance.

Occupational location is a key factor in the lack of health insurance for Mexican-origin women, in that many of these women are located in low-wage job sectors. There are also other factors that influence their lack of coverage, however. Marital status, poverty status, education status, and levels of acculturation correlate with health insurance status. For example, a married woman is more likely to have health insurance through her husband's employment. If she speaks Spanish and identifies herself as a Mexican rather than as Mexican American or Chicana, she is less likely to have health insurance. Finally, both her educational level and whether she is above or below the federal poverty level will greatly influence whether she has financial access to health care through the voluntary health insurance market. In addition, culturally defined gender roles in the household may limit Mexican-origin women's employment prospects, as do life-cycle decisions such as pregnancy and child rearing. These decisions can interrupt employment and affect a woman's decision to work. The ability of recently immigrated women to adapt to the institutional environment and bureaucratic health-care system of the United States also places real constraints on access to public and private health insurance. Thus, for Mexican-origin women, the issue of health-care access goes beyond a simple model linked to employment and encompasses broader social issues that are defined by their immigrant status, marital status, and other factors.[17] Recognizing these gender differences is an important step in targeting health coverage strategies for uninsured and underinsured Mexican-origin women.

The PPACA tries to provide for women and single-woman families that may fall through the cracks of paying for insurance. Table 17 shows the considerations the PPACA has for women and children. One example

Table 17. Coverage of Women and Children under PPACA

TYPE OF COVERAGE	WOMEN	CHILDREN
Increased coverage	Same as adult men	Can be covered under parents' insurance until age 26
Waiting period for documented immigrants and access to Medicaid	Some states allow pregnant women to waive the five-year waiting period	Some states allow children to waive the five-year waiting period
Coverage for preexisting conditions	Coverage required under PPACA	Coverage required under PPACA
Preventative care (a sample)	*Well-woman visits, mammograms, breastfeeding support and supplies, IPV support and counseling, pregnancy screening and counseling	Depression screening (teens), autism screening (newborns), immunizations, obesity screening and counseling

Sources: Healthcare.gov, National Immigration Law Center; HHS.gov, "Affordable Care Act Rules on Expanding Access to Preventive Services for Women," website: http://www.hhs.gov/healthcare/; CMS.gov, "Center for Consumer Information and Insurance Oversight," website: http://www.healthcare.gov/; National Immigration Law Center, "Immigrants and the Affordable Care Act," website: http://www.nilc.org/.
* Eight additional preventative-care measures have been added specifically for women to meet the health needs of women and reduce disparities in health between men and women (e.g., women are more likely to pay more out of pocket and avoid/delay care).

of the way the PPACA tries to provide for the specific needs of women is through the increased amount of preventative care services for pregnancy and breastfeeding supplies women can receive. In addition to helping women specifically, teenagers will receive depression screenings in order to provide support for this common effect of puberty. All of these changes are aimed at satisfying the insurance needs of particular subpopulations and emphasize preventative care instead of expensive emergency-care services.

Undocumented Mexican-Origin Immigrants

A small yet important group within the immigrant population is composed of undocumented immigrants of Mexican origin. Of the thirty million Mexican Americans in the United States, twelve million are foreign born. Currently, an estimated eleven million undocumented immigrants reside in the United States. Of these, 62 percent are from Mexico. The state with the highest number of undocumented immigrants is California, where 24 percent of all U.S. undocumented immigrants reside.

Mexico is the country of origin of more than half of all undocumented immigrants. While the term "Latino/a" is used to describe undocumented immigrants in some reports, approximately 80 percent of all Latino/a undocumented immigrants are of Mexican origin.[18] Therefore, the use of the Latino/a ethnic designation may not be very useful when it comes to describing undocumented immigrants. We recommend population-specific terms that are based on country of origin. The fact that Mexicans are overwhelmingly represented within the Latino/a undocumented immigrant group can be seen in table 18.

Table 18.   Undocumented Latino/a Immigrants by Country of Origin and Population Size, 2009

COUNTRY OF ORIGIN	U.S. POPULATION SIZE
Mexico	6,650,000
El Salvador	530,000
Guatemala	480,000
Honduras	320,000
Ecuador	170,000
Brazil	150,000

Source: M. Hoefer, N. Rytina, and B. C. Baker, "Estimates of the Unauthorized Immigrant Population Residing in the United States: January 2009," *DHS Office of Immigration Statistics, Population Estimates* (2010): 1–8.

Table 19. Undocumented Immigrant Population in Four Southwestern States

STATE OF RESIDENCE	POPULATION
California	2,600,000
Texas	1,680,000
Arizona	460,000
Nevada	260,000

Source: M. Hoefer, N. Rytina, and B. C. Baker, "Estimates of the Unauthorized Immigrant Population Residing in the United States: January 2009," DHS Office of Immigration Statistics, Population Estimates (2010): 1–8.

The largest portion of the undocumented population is located in the Southwest; a state-by-state breakdown is provided in table 19. One can easily understand how the proximity of Mexico, as well as the large Mexican-origin population in these states, serves as a magnet for undocumented immigration. However, location and ethnic concentration are insufficient to explain the overrepresentation of undocumented immigrants in the Southwest. A primary reason that undocumented workers from Mexico are lured to the Southwest is the large demand for low-wage labor in service-sector industries and agriculture. This "pull" to the United States is further exacerbated by the "push" from Mexico's less-developed economy, where the average daily wage is significantly lower than that paid in the United States. For example, the Mexican minimum wage in U.S. dollars is $4.45 per day compared to the U.S. minimum wage, which is $7.25 per hour, or $58.00 per day before taxes.[19]

The fact that many undocumented workers are employed in low-wage sectors of the U.S. economy has direct implications for their access to adequate health care and health insurance. Most are employed in sectors that offer no health insurance to employees; thus, they have no access to health care except for emergency services. Moreover, because they have immigrated without documentation, most avoid seeking health care except in emergencies for fear of detection and deportation by U.S. Citizenship and Immigration Services, formerly referred to as the Immigration and Naturalization Service (INS) or La Migra.

According to a study by the Project HOPE Center for Health Affairs, this low rate of coverage presents problems such as a lower use of private physician services and a greater reliance on local clinics and health centers for primary care needs, compared to legal immigrants. In addition, the second most likely site of care for undocumented immigrants is the emergency room, which is a costly alternative for treatment. This study also suggests that because undocumented immigrants have high rates of poverty, they may have lower expectations for care and be unable to pay for treatments, which may explain their underutilization of health-care services. Unlike other large Latino/a subpopulations, such as Puerto Rican and Cuban Americans, the issue of legal status is an important health-care policy issue for Mexican-origin immigrants. This differential treatment is due to the proximity of Mexico to the United States, the historical exploitation of cheap Mexican labor in the Southwest and elsewhere, and the regional concentration of undocumented Mexican immigrants in states such as California and Arizona. Even though the number of undocumented immigrants is relatively small compared to legal Mexican immigrants and Mexican Americans, the continued presence of undocumented Mexican-origin persons and the political backlash of the white electorate require special consideration in addressing access issues for this group.

El Instituto Nacional de Salud Pública, or the Mexican Institute of Public Health, has tried to implement a binational coverage program for Mexican immigrants in the United States. This program, called Salud Migrante, has been a pilot project carried out in North Carolina and Washington States. Salud Migrante allows Mexican guest workers to receive emergency coverage in the United States and nonemergency care in Mexico. The Mexican government sends payments to community clinics in the United States to support immigrants covered under Salud Migrante. This coverage would reduce the financial burden of uninsured immigrants on the United States' emergency facilities. Hopefully this program will allow undocumented and uninsured Mexican Americans to integrate more easily into the U.S. health-care system.

Table 20 compares the type of coverage an individual can expect to receive under the PPACA based on their immigration status in the United States. The PPACA extends policy changes to citizens and documented immigrants, but the new law mostly excludes undocumented immigrants, who are not allowed to utilize the public health-care programs. This law has a large effect on Latino populations, since Latino immigrants are more likely to be undocumented than are other immigrant populations.

The restrictions on undocumented immigrants to receive health insurance through the PPACA places even more importance on comprehensive

Table 20. Immigration Status and Access to Health Care under PPACA

	NATIVE-BORN/ NATURALIZED CITIZENS	DOCUMENTED IMMIGRANTS	UNDOCUMENTED IMMIGRANTS
Amount of federal coverage	Full	Limited	None
Individual mandate	Applies	Applies	Does not apply
Participation in state insurance exchanges	Allowed	*Allowed	Not allowed
Medicaid/Medicare/ Children's Health Insurance Program eligibility	Eligible	Eligible with waiting period	Only eligible for emergency services
Waiting period for Medicaid	None	†Five-year residency	N/A

Source: National Immigration Law Center website: http://www.nilc.org/. Last updated March 2013.
* Allowed to participate in a "Qualified Health Plan" (QHP).
† Some states may waive the waiting period for pregnant women or children (applies to SCHIP as well).

immigration reform. When the first edition of this book was published, a new immigration reform bill that would create a pathway for undocumented immigrants to become U.S. citizens was up for debate in Congress. Additionally, President Obama restricted the deportation of undocumented children and undocumented immigrants who entered the United States before they were sixteen years old. In addition to other restrictions on deportation, these Executive Actions, as these were called, provided some reprieve for undocumented immigrants in the United States. Immigration reform will be an important factor influencing Latinos/as and their access to healthcare in the coming years.

The Role of Minority Health-Care Professionals in Access to Care

The health of minority populations will continue to lag behind as long as we continue to be underrepresented in the health professions. Mexican American communities have a dearth of providers. This proves to be a deterrent to access for many potential health care consumers. . . . The perspective of the Latino physician and scientist, at the bedside and at the lab bench, is crucial for the well-being of the entire community. (Francisco G., MD, 35)

The smallness of the pool of minority health-care professionals (e.g., physicians, nurses, dentists, and physical therapists) is another significant issue affecting health-care access. The shortage of Latino health-care professionals limits access to health care for the Mexican-origin population because minority health professionals overwhelmingly serve in their communities. Most of these communities are poor and are underserved because of the low ratio of health professionals in this population. According to a Council on Graduate Medical Education report entitled "Minorities in Medicine," Latino health-care professionals are important because they bridge the gap between the culture of the minority group and that of health-care service providers. The report concluded:

1. Minority physicians practice in medically underserved areas at almost twice the rate of nonminority physicians.
2. Minority patients were four times more likely than majority white patients to receive their health-care services from nonwhite physicians than from white physicians.
3. Compared to the service areas for non-Latino physicians, there are twice as many Latino residents in the areas where Latino physicians practice.
4. Latino physicians provide health care to three times as many Latino patients as do non-Latino physicians.[20]

Thus, Latino physicians, like other minority physicians, provide Latinos with greater access to care. They not only locate their practices where there are more Latino residents but also serve more Latino patients than do their non-Latino physician counterparts.

Given the documented importance of the role of minority physicians, the **American Association of Medical Colleges** (AAMC) in 1991 launched a major program known as "Project 3000 by 2000." Its goal was to increase the percentage of minority matriculation in **allopathic** medical schools to 19 percent of total **matriculants**. This percentage reflects the proportion of minorities in the total U.S. population in the year 2000. The number of minority medical students needed in these medical schools to reach parity within the U.S. population by 2000 was 3,000.[21] Unfortunately, the AAMC's goal was not met, primarily because of a strong

Table 21. National Medical School Applicant Pool, 2011: Selected Groups

APPLICANTS	APPLIED	ACCEPTED	ENROLLED
White	23,957	11,577	11,060
African American	3,215	1,231	1,182
Mexican American	816	446*	426*

Source: Association of American Medical Colleges, Diversity in Medical Education: Facts and Figures 2012 (Washington, DC: Association of American Medical Colleges, 2012).
* This number was available for the Latino racial/ethnicity group only. The term "Latino" includes Cuban, Mexican American, Puerto Rican, other Latino, and multiple Latino.

anti-affirmative-action movement that swept the United States during the 1990s. For example, in California, **Proposition 209** ended affirmative action in all public institutions, particularly the University of California system. The **Hopwood decision** in Texas also targeted affirmative-action programs in higher education, lowering the number of minority applicants to medical and other health professional schools. However, the scope of affirmative-action programs in higher education is still debated through different Supreme Court rulings. In 2003, the *Grutter v. Bollinger* case set the precedent that affirmative action programs could be in place if the racial status of a college applicant was but one factor used to determine enrollment eligibility in the interest of maintaining diversity within the student body. How this decision has been implemented in school admission programs is still being debated as of the writing of this book (see *Fisher v. University of Texas at Austin*).

In the case of Mexican American physicians, the minority underrepresentation resulting from attacks on affirmative action programs becomes immediately apparent early on in the **educational pipeline**. Few medical-school applicants are of Mexican descent and even fewer are accepted into medical schools. Although other minority groups face the same situation, it is disproportionately severe for Mexican-origin applicants given the small number of applicants to begin with (see table 21).[22]

The percentage of Latina women in medical schools is growing but at a lower rate than that of African American women. While in 2011 African American women represented 62 percent of the total African American matriculants in medical school, Mexican American women follow a similar pattern as white non-Latina women with respect to representation, with women constituting 47.4 percent of Mexican American matriculants

Table 22.   Matriculated Medical Students, 2011: Selected Racial/Ethnic Groups

RACE/ETHNICITY	MEN	WOMEN	TOTAL
African American	445 (38%)	737 (62%)	1,182
Mexican American	224 (53%)	202 (47%)	426
White non-Latino	6,252 (57%)	4,808 (43%)	11,060
Total (all groups)	6,921 (57%)	5,747 (45%)	12,668

Source: Association of American Medical Colleges, *Diversity in Medical Education: Facts & Figures 2012* (Washington, DC: Association of American Medical Colleges, 2012).

and 43.5 percent of white non-Latino matriculants. As illustrated in table 22, there is a clear need to increase the number of both Mexican American men and women in the medical profession. Table 22 also illustrates the crisis in meeting the goal of "Project 3000 by 2000." By 2011, there were only 1,608 African American and Mexican American first-year students in U.S. medical schools, far below the stated goal of 3,000. Even with the support of the AAMC, the most powerful voice of U.S. medical colleges, meeting the needs of minority communities has not been possible to achieve through the educational pipeline.

The University of California Programs in Medical Education (UC PRIME) is an important model for tackling the problem of underrepresentation in medical schools. The UC PRIME focus on educating medical professionals who can work with California's underserved rural and urban communities. The different UC medical campuses have developed specific educational and training programs based on the subpopulations they serve. For example, the UC PRIME at Irvine focuses specifically on the needs of Latino communities and tries to train medical professionals to serve this community. The UC PRIME was first implemented across the University of California system in 2007, although the UC Irvine program first admitted students in 2004. Hopefully these programs will be able to provide better culturally and regionally competent care to Latinos and other groups in need of sensitive health-care professionals.

Concluding Thoughts

A number of issues affect the Mexican-origin population's access to health care in the United States. Foremost is the problem of financial access. This problem is intrinsically tied to occupational location, which determines the income level of this subpopulation and whether or not they have access to private or publicly subsidized health insurance coverage. However, certain segments of the Mexican-origin population are more severely constrained by issues of financial access than are others. For example, senior citizens, undocumented immigrants, and women have special situations that interfere with their ability to effectively use both public and private health insurance.

In the past the complexity of the U.S. health-care financing system, which elevated private health insurance above universal coverage for all individuals, created a policy dilemma for those of Mexican origin. The passage of the PPACA will hopefully help address the needs of this disproportionately uninsured group. As the PPACA is fully implemented and immigration reform is considered in the United States, the U.S. Mexican-origin population may start to see their health-care needs met more fully.

A final important point with regard to access to health care is the shortage of Mexican-origin health-care professionals available to serve this population. As illustrated by the case of Mexican American physicians, without aggressive outreach efforts and early educational intervention the persistence of low numbers of medical applicants and graduates will continue. An excellent model for addressing this educational issue is provided by UC PRIME.

Discussion Exercises

1. What problems does the Mexican-origin community face in regard to financial access to health insurance?

2. What model has proven useful for examining predictors of health-care access and utilization?

3. What are the differences between publicly subsidized and private health insurance programs?

4. How does the lack of health insurance coverage affect the health status of the Mexican American population?

5. How does immigrant status affect one's ability to obtain health care and insurance in the United States? Discuss in particular the difficulty of enrolling in public health insurance programs.

6. What is the relationship between occupational location and financial access to adequate health-care services?

7. Why is it important to have parity in terms of minority health-care professionals? What role does the education system play in reaching parity and increasing the pool of minority health-care professionals?

Notes

1. AHCCCS, the Arizona Health Care Cost Containment System, is the Arizona Medicaid-funded health program for the medically indigent.

2. L. Gelberg, R. M. Andersen, and B. D. Leake., "The Behavioral Model for Vulnerable Populations: Application to Medical Care Use and Outcomes for Homeless People," *Health Services Research* 34, no. 6 (2000): 1273–1302; J. A. Stein, R. M. Andersen, and L. Gelberg, "Applying the Gelberg-Andersen Behavioral Model for Vulnerable Populations to Health Services Utilization in Homeless Women," *Journal of Health Psychology* 12, no. 5 (2007): 791–804.

3. S. J. Williams and P. R. Torrens, *Introduction to Health Services*, 2nd ed. (New York: Wiley, 1984), 420.

4. J. Park and J. S. Buechner, "Race, Ethnicity, and Access to Health Care, Rhode Island," *Journal of Health and Social Policy* 9, no. 1 (1997).

5. American Community Survey, S2701: Health Insurance Coverage Status, *2009 American Community Survey 1-Year Estimates*, retrieved on November 19, 2010, from http://factfinder.census.gov/.

6. Ibid.

7. *Comparison of the Prevalence of Uninsured Persons from the National Health Interview Survey and the Current Population Survey, January–April 2014* (National Center for Health Statistics, U.S. Census Bureau, September 2014).

8. Social Security Administration website: http://www.socialsecurity.gov/, search keyword SSI.

9. Reference for Business. "Medicare and Medicaid" in *Encyclopedia of Business*, 2nd ed. Retrieved on November 19, 2010, from http://www.referenceforbusiness.com/.

10. Ibid.

11. "What Is Medicare?" available from the Medicare website: http://www.medicare.gov/.

12. Ibid.

13. Department of Health and Human Services, *Health Insurance Marketplace: Summary Enrollment Report for the Period: October 1, 2013–February 19, 2014*, ASPE Issue Brief, May 1, 2014.

14. President Obama's success in the 2012 election was in part due to the strong Latino vote he received in vital swing states. Latinos, as the fastest growing population

in the United States, with a 43 percent increase in the Latino population between 2000 and 2010, have become an important political force. Additionally, Latinos are a young population, with two million new Latinos reaching the voting age between 2008 and 2012. In addition, Latinos as a group have increased their voter mobilization in recent elections. Latinos made up 10 percent of the voters in the 2012 election (up from 9 percent in the 2008 presidential election).

15. J. Guyer and C. Mann, "Employed but Not Insured: A State-by-State Analysis of the Number of Low-Income Working Parents Who Lack Health Insurance," 3; available from the Center on Budget and Policy Priorities website: http://www.cbpp.org/.

16. "Heart disease, diabetes and cancer of the breast, colon, and cervix are the leading causes of death for Latinas living in the United States" (14). "These diseases are most likely to impact these women in their middle to elderly years. . . . For example, Mexican-born women represent 48 percent of all cancer deaths in the state of Texas and have 37 percent higher 28-day myocardial infarction mortality rates when compared to non-Latino white counterparts" (16, 17). "Other research has shown that Mexican women in the Southwest have two times the rate of cervical cancer than that of their non-Latino counterparts, which could be linked to the fact that a higher percentage of these women speak predominantly Spanish" (19). "Also, less acculturated women over 50 years of age were much less likely to have had a mammogram" (20). A. de la Torre et al., "The Health Insurance Status of Latinas: A Population at Risk," *Journal of Border Health* 4 (1999): 1–24.

17. A. de la Torre et al., "The Health Insurance Status of U.S. Latino Women: A Profile from the 1982–84 Hispanic HHANES," *American Journal of Public Health* 86, no. 4 (April 1996): 534.

18. Although the study from which this information was taken uses the term "Latino," the vast majority of the population under study were of Mexican origin; C. L. Schu et al., *California's Undocumented Latino Immigrants: A Report on Access to Health Care Services* (Bethesda, MD: The Project HOPE Center for Health Affairs, 1999), 35.

19. This information is for January 2010. The Mexican minimum wage varies depending on geographical region. Mexperience website: http://www.mexperience.com/.

20. D. L. Libby, Z. Zhou, and D. A. Kindig, "Will Minority Physician Supply Meet U.S. Needs?" *Health Affairs* 16, no. 4 (1997): 205–14; Council on Graduate Medical Education, "Minorities in Medicine," May 1998.

21. Association of American Medical Colleges (AAMC) *Project 3000 by 2000 Progress to Date: Year Four Progress Report* (Washington, DC: AAMC, Division of Community and Minority Programs, 1996), 1.

22. Presentation by Jordon Cohen, MD, president of the AAMC at the AAMC Conference, Washington, DC, October 1999. In 1997, 796 Mexican Americans applied

to medical schools in the United States. Approximately half of these were accepted and enrolled. However, since 1991, the number of Mexican American medical school applicants has decreased by almost 14 percent. This decline is directly related to the cutbacks in affirmative-action programs in California and Texas, where a large number of Mexican-origin students reside.

Suggested Readings

Glaser, W. A. *Health Insurance in Practice.* San Francisco and Oxford: Jossey-Bass, 1991.

Hernández, D. J. *Children of Immigrants: Health, Adjustment, and Public Assistance.* Washington, DC: National Academy Press, 1999.

Kass, B. L., R. M. Weinick, and A. C. Monheit. *Racial and Ethnic Differences in Health, 1996.* MEPS Chartbook No. 2. Available from the Agency for Health Care Policy Research website: www.meps.ahcpr.gov/.

Medicare website: www.medicare.gov.

Staff of the Washington Post. *Landmark: The Inside Story of America's New Health Care Law and What it Means for Us All.* New York: PublicAffairs, 2010.

U.S. Bureau of the Census. *Health Insurance Coverage, 1997.* Current Population Reports, Series P60–202. Washington, DC: U.S. Bureau of the Census, September 1998.

Williams, S. J., and P. R. Torrens. *Introduction to Health Services.* 2nd ed. New York: Wiley, 1984.

Chapter 5

Cultural Competency in Health-Care Services

"My Doctor Doesn't Care"

It's like there's a clash there somewhere, and I don't know if it's cultural or what it is. I don't know if doctors understand how to deal with people who don't speak the language or Mexicans from Mexico or Chicanos or Chicanas. I don't know if there's a cultural clash or what it is exactly, but they tend to be a bit brisk at times or they shun people off like, "shut up." . . . (Marco G., 28)

Marco illustrates the frustration of many Mexican Americans who feel that they are not being provided with culturally competent health care. This frustration may result from the lack of health-care professionals who have Spanish language skills, a health-care professional's use of negative stereotypes when addressing patients in a clinical setting, or the general lack of cultural sensitivity in the diagnosis or treatment of an illness. This chapter will focus on the importance of both linguistic and cultural competency in providing quality health care to the Mexican-origin population. Given the introductory nature of this book, we will highlight the current issues and debates surrounding this topic. However, we recognize that this is a new and rapidly emerging field. Over the years, advocacy from patients and minority health-care professionals has pushed this issue to the forefront of the national health-care debate.

Linguistic Competency: A Significant Component of Cultural Competency

It was important to my mother that her doctor was Mexican or Latino. To her it made a difference because I can remember being seven or eight years old and translating what the doctor was saying. At the time I didn't think it was a big deal, but now that I look back I think that it was kind of hard on me because I felt that I had to clearly state what he was saying to her and vice versa. I don't know how well of a job I did at that time. That's why it was important to her to make sure that she had a doctor that could speak Spanish, that was bilingual. (Ana M., 26)

Ana, like many children of Mexican immigrants, experienced firsthand the dilemma of translating for her parents during visits to the doctor's office. In the absence of bilingual medical staff or an adult interpreter, she was the only means of communication between her mother and the clinician. Ana's childhood experiences illustrate the frustrations and fears many children from Mexican immigrant families experience in translating for their parents when health problems that require direct medical intervention arise.

Unfortunately, many children of Mexican immigrants are still placed in the awkward position of seeking the best medical treatment for their families by acting as a linguistic bridge to the dominant culture and language of the United States. Yet given the sophistication of medical information, few children are able to effectively understand and synthesize it, which can result in potentially dangerous miscommunication between physician and patient. Therein lies the inherent weakness in relying on these young bridges to meet the linguistic needs of this large Spanish-speaking community. In states such as California that have large Latino populations, the need to provide linguistically competent health care to Spanish-speaking immigrants has become a major force in restructuring how health care is delivered. The goals are to minimize the need for family members to act as interpreters for relatives in the delivery of health-care services and to increase the delivery of information through either professional interpreters on site or trained bilingual health-care professionals.

Linguistic competency is critical to granting health-care access to many Mexican immigrants. Linguistic competency, for most health-care professionals, is defined as the availability of health-care information and services in the language of the patient. The key is whether health-care professionals can communicate with Spanish-speaking clients in a way that results in improved health outcomes for the clients and lower costs for the providers of these services. As recent Mexican immigrants become the dominant segment of the Mexican-origin population, the need for bilingual health professionals will increase.

Newly arrived immigrants generally have little education, do not speak English, and are less acculturated. Therefore, they are at greater risk of encountering barriers to health care when they are not provided with linguistically competent health-care providers.[1] Monolingual Spanish speakers are also at the greatest risk of not obtaining health care because of their lower rate of private health insurance coverage compared to bilingual Spanish-English and monolingual English speakers.[2] Thus, language plays an important role in enabling recent Mexican immigrants to access health care in the United States.

Linguistic competency is an essential component of cultural competency for the Mexican-origin population given its demographic profile and recent immigrant status. California's model for contracting managed-care plans for the Medi-Cal (California's state Medicaid program) beneficiaries has been relatively successful in addressing the linguistic competency issue. To address the state's multicultural health-care needs, it was determined that the linguistic needs of non-English-speaking health plan members must be met. Therefore, California requires that health plans contracting to serve the Medi-Cal-eligible population must translate health plan materials into the language of non-English-speaking clients and provide twenty-four-hour interpreter services. A lesson learned from the California experience is that the first step in meeting the cultural needs of immigrant populations is incorporating linguistic services into the health-care system.[3]

Beyond the issue of translation and interpreter services within health-care settings is the profile of the medical staff at the site. The California experience also highlights the need for incentives to hire more Latino and Mexican-origin physicians within the Medi-Cal delivery system. As many of these providers share both language and cultural values with the patients they serve, they are better equipped to understand the cultural nuances of the largely monolingual and bilingual Mexican-origin population. Unfortunately, the paucity of Latino physicians in the United States has resulted in a significant shortage of bilingual and culturally competent health-care providers. As discussed in chapter 4, the prospect of meeting the growing demand for bilingual and bicultural doctors in the near future appears bleak. As illustrated in table 23, Mexican-origin students constituted just under 3 percent of medical-school graduates in 2010.

Focusing on Spanish-language competency alone as the defining characteristic of linguistic competency is problematic, however. Since language is symbolic of the broader cultural experience of Mexican Americans and Mexican immigrants, understanding the cultural nuances and idiosyncratic belief structures of this group is critical to interpreting language.

Table 23. Ethnic Background of Medical School Graduates, 2011

ETHNIC BACKGROUND	# OF GRADUATES
African American	1,129
Native American/Alaskan Native	135
Mexican American	456
Puerto Rican	357
Other Latino	422
Asian/Pacific Islander	3,816
Non-Latino white	10,733

Source: Association of American Medical Colleges, *Diversity in Medical Education: Facts & Figures 2012* (Washington, DC: Association of American Medical Colleges, 2012).

Thus, a broader definition of competency should include an understanding of Mexican folklore and health.

The Impact of Mexican Folklore, Language, and Health

> The only times that we ended up in the hospital or in the doctor's office is when it was an extreme emergency. All other things, such as the upset stomachs, the burns, the cuts, the scrapes, were taken care of by herbs, teas, and home remedies, which my mother had great knowledge of. She was very well versed in the folkloric healing caused by, for example, el mal de ojo, susto, and empacho. (Gracie S., 46)

Gracie illustrates how low-income immigrant families often rely on a family member to provide treatment for childhood and family illnesses. In many Mexican immigrant families, the health-care providers are mothers who learned through their kinship ties about Mexican folklore (i.e., the beliefs, attitudes, behaviors drawn from traditional sociocultural experiences) and illnesses and remedies. This is further illustrated by Gracie's childhood experience with the mumps:

> We ended up getting mumps all at the same time. There were nine of us and seven of us ended up with the mumps. This was a struggle for my mother because we all had high fevers. She didn't have money for pain medication or fever medication; she just knew how to do things according to how she was raised. She knew that the discomfort of mumps was alleviated by applying heat, so she sautéed tomatoes and wrapped them around

our cheeks. And she would sauté tomatoes and put them on the bottom of our feet. (Gracie S., 46)

Gracie's family experience with the mumps illustrates why a clinician would need to not only have a command of the Spanish language but also have some familiarity with cultural interpretations of illnesses and traditional treatments used by Mexican immigrants. Often linguistic competency is viewed solely as the ability of a clinician to speak to patients in their native language as well as in English. However, linguistic competency must go beyond translation by bilingual medical personnel. It must include health promotion and educational materials that are culturally appropriate to and at the literacy level of the patient. Given the low educational levels of many Mexican immigrants, linguistically appropriate material needs to use suitable means of communication for patients to fully understand treatments for themselves and their families. This may require medical providers to be sensitive to regional dialects of Spanish as well as the use and knowledge of idiomatic expressions and cultural beliefs of diseases to convey information about certain health disorders. For example, illnesses may be expressed using spiritual and folkloric aspects of Mexican culture rather than through explicit reference to actual diseases. Emotional and physiological responses to these perceived illnesses can be understood only if the health provider is both linguistically and culturally aware of these beliefs. According to Margarita Kay:

> Many health problems have names that are readily recognizable across cultures. In the American and Mexican West, however, some of these illnesses have old-fashioned names that were once the established terms for specific diseases but which are seen today simply as symptoms by biomedicine ("fever" is one example). . . . Folk illnesses, called "Mexican diseases" by Mexican Americans because "American doctors don't believe in them," have other seemingly obsolete names.[4]

Table 24 lists symptomatic diseases that do not have exact English translations or counterparts, illustrating the cultural and idiomatic specificity of Mexican diseases. Such folkloric illnesses are embedded in cultural interpretations that may result in patient-clinician misunderstanding if the medical staff is unaware of them. The situation is further complicated when a patient treats an illness with folkloric remedies. Within the cultural parameters of Mexican folklore are herbal remedies used

Table 24.   Some Common Folkloric Diseases and Their Treatments

DISEASE	DEFINITION	TREATMENT
Empacho	Swollen belly resulting from massage by a *sobadora* or from undigested food.	Drinking herbal teas such as *yerba buena* (peppermint) or *manzanilla* (chamomile).
Espanto	*Susto* or fright caused by seeing a ghost or being awakened suddenly; more serious than *susto.*	Retrieving one's soul, *limpia,* or house blessing.
Mal de ojo	Often mistranslated as "the evil eye," this is "illness caused by staring"; results when infants or children receive more attention than usual; can result in restlessness, vomiting, or fever.	Rubbing an egg over the child as prayers are recited using a special charm or amulet.
Mollera caída	In infants, this represents a fallen fontanel, which may be a result of dehydration.	Wetting the baby's head with warm water, soaping the soft spot, then gently pushing up on the palate while pulling the hairs on the soft spot.
Pasmo	Swellings and skin eruptions resulting from rapid chilling of the body following excessive activity or bleeding.	N/A
Pujos	In infants, grunting or straining as a result of contact with menstruating women or persons who have recently had sexual intercourse.	N/A

Sources: E. Ávila and J. Parker, *Woman Who Glows in the Dark* (New York: Jeremy P. Tarcher/Putnam, 1999); R. T. Trotter and J. A. Chavira, *Curanderismo, Mexican American Folk Healing* (Athens: University of Georgia Press, 1997).

for treatment of a disease, as illustrated in table 24. **Curanderas/os** (folk healers) use many treatments, both medicinal and ritual, to help people recover from the illnesses listed in the table and others. Two common treatments are *limpias* (cleanings) and *pláticas* (conversations). A limpia is a spiritual cleansing used to heal emotional trauma that may or may not be manifesting physically. This treatment often involves sweeping an egg or bundles of herbs over the body to "cleanse a person's energy." This may be done in combination with praying or chanting. Pláticas, according to

Elena Ávila, a Mexican American curandera, are "heart-to-heart talks" that perform the functions of culturally sensitive counseling. Pláticas help the curandera and patient to discover together the possible causes of an illness and can be curative in themselves. These two types of treatment are used, in various forms, to address a range of emotional/spiritual and physical illnesses. Because of a lack of health insurance, it is not uncommon for Mexican-origin persons, especially low-income immigrants, to seek alternative treatments or to delay treatment for a disease until a medical crisis emerges.[5]

Anthropologists have conducted much of the research on Mexican folkloric illnesses and treatment, and there is very little documentation of the extent to which folkloric practices are used within the Mexican-origin community. Again, a lack of financial access to health care may lead to greater reliance on kinship ties to diagnose and treat the symptoms of an illness. Although the documented evidence to date provides little support for widespread use of traditional Mexican healers (including curanderas, **parteras**, or **sobadoras**), knowledgeable family members may often act as substitutes for these healers.

Recent health-care literature is instructive on how cultural competency can be integrated into the health-care delivery system. This literature further develops the idea of incorporating individual cultural beliefs and practices as mediating factors in diagnosing and treating patients. This broader definition provides an opportunity for improving access to and the quality of health care for the Mexican-origin population.

Cultural Competency: Implications for the Mexican-Origin Population

Cultural Competency is a process that requires individuals and systems to develop and expand their ability to know about, be sensitive to, and have respect for cultural diversity. The result of this process should be an increased awareness, acceptance, valuing, and utilization of and an openness to learn from general and health-related beliefs, practices, traditions, languages, religions, histories, and current needs of individuals and the cultural groups to which they belong. Essential to cultural competency is appropriate and effective communication. This requires the willingness to listen and learn from members of diverse cultures and the provision of services and information in appropriate languages, at appropriate comprehension and literacy levels, and in the context of individuals' cultural health beliefs and practices.[6]

During the last decade the body of literature focusing on cultural competency and access to quality health care has increased. As the nation's minority population continues to grow, the lack of minority trained health professionals and the general ignorance of cultural issues will continue to create barriers to health-care access for this population. Given the individual health-care risks and the costs associated with limited access, cultural competency has moved from the margins of the health-care debates to the forefront.

In the area of substance-abuse prevention there is a significant body of literature describing interventions that are sensitive to ethnic, racial, gender, regional, and class differences within targeted populations. A significant amount of this work has focused on the Latino community in general without examining inter- and intra-group differences, which limits its usefulness for the Mexican-origin population. However, research suggests that health-care providers who have a clear understanding of differences between Latino groups will be more effective in developing cost-effective programs for them.

Another rich source of information is the literature on mental health. Yet, despite the significance of this work in isolating unique cultural behaviors of distinct Latino subpopulations, this literature often ignores the historical experience of immigrants. Without an understanding of how Mexican immigrants enter the United States and acculturate, only a superficial understanding of their culture is possible. For many Mexican immigrants, the way they enter the United States influences how they construct their identity and minority group status. This is illustrated by the following interview with Martín:

> I came here when I was nine. . . . My mother was back in Mexico. After my grandmother died I felt like I didn't belong there [in Mexico] anymore so I wanted to get away and I was sent over [to live] with my aunt in the United States. I was closer to my grandmother than I was to my mother. . . . In the beginning it was tough because there was a language barrier. I didn't know how to speak a word of English and there was no bilingual program. I had a cousin who had the same classes and translated what was going on in the classroom for me, but it was hard to pick up the language. All of the kids

made fun of you and called you wetback and *mojado* because you couldn't speak the language and they knew you were from a different country. So it was hard. (Martín G., 31)

Martín illustrates the ambivalent feelings that Mexican immigrants often have about living in the United States. Even though his "push factors" (reasons for leaving Mexico) were personal, related to the loss of his beloved grandmother, his reception into the United States was less than hospitable. His ethnic identity and his limited English skills caused him to suffer the discrimination that many Mexican immigrants have experienced in the Southwest. Thus, his identity has been shaped by his ethnicity and the discrimination he has faced. Unfortunately, the literature on public health glosses over this social construction of ethnic identity and the multiple dimensions of cultural and individual identity.

Martín's case also illustrates another important factor in framing culturally competent interventions, namely, recognizing the immigrant status of the Mexican-origin population. Immigrant status affects not only language preference (level of Spanish or English proficiency) but also the relative importance of cultural practices from Mexico. For example, much of the literature that focuses on positive birth outcomes (for example, low infant mortality) analyzes data of recent Mexican immigrant women. Studies by David Hayes Bautista and colleagues illustrate well the differences between Mexican immigrant women and Mexican Americans of later generations.[7] Generally, immigrant women are likely to adhere to more rigid class and male-female cultural norms, including those relating to health-care issues such as the use of traditional home remedies to self-treat an ailment or condition. Research by Raffaelli and Ontai (2001, 2004) strongly suggests that young Mexican-origin women and men are particularly socialized by their parents to maintain traditional gender roles in social relations and cultural norms.[8]

As children of immigrants become acculturated through their new educational and social milieus, perceptions and health-care practices begin to change. For young Mexican American women in particular there is significant historical evidence of increased intergenerational conflict as young women develop a new sense of social identity and placement within the larger society. This legacy of intergenerational conflict is best illustrated in Vicki Ruiz' analysis of Mexican-origin women in Los Angeles in the 1930s.

Conflicts erupted within families as young Latinas attempted to emulate the Hollywood standard of the day in behavior and dress:

> Within families, young women, perhaps more than their brothers, were expected to uphold certain standards. Indeed, Chicano/a social scientists have generally portrayed women as "the 'glue' that keeps the Chicano family together" and as the guardians of "traditional culture." Parents, therefore, often assumed what they perceived as their unquestionable prerogative to regulate the actions and attitudes of their adolescent daughters. Teenagers, on the other hand, did not always acquiesce in the boundaries set down for them by their elders. Intergenerational tension flared along several fronts.[9]

In many respects, children of immigrants create blended or bicultural identities that may challenge traditional roles while symbolically still supporting traditional markers of ethnic identity such as language and religious practices. Biculturalism within immigrant and ethnic groups is not unique to the Mexican-origin population. Dual identity and cultural practices are seen in most Latino/a groups, including Dominicans, Puerto Ricans, and Cubans.[10] Understanding the cultural identity of Mexican Americans and other Latino subgroups is a first step in appropriately defining culturally specific health-care practices and interventions.

Microaggressions

While many minorities in America are familiar with overt racism, such as ethnic slurs or systematic discrimination against a particular group (e.g., schools segregated by race and/or ethnicity), more subtle forms of racism may be unfamiliar. While overt racism may be perceived as largely a thing of the past in America, racial microaggressions, or subtle, sometimes unintentional forms of racism, are extremely common. Racial microaggressions occur when, typically, a member of the majority makes every day comments that marginalize or devalue the racial experiences of minority groups. For example, a white person telling a Latino man that they "don't see skin color" devalues the Latino's ethnic or racial identity.

While microaggressions are very commonplace, and are often unnoticed or even denied by the person who committed them, they can still have a significant impact on minority individuals. Microaggressions often cause minority individuals to question themselves: "Did that actually happen?" "Should I say something?" "Were they trying to be racist, or was it a coincidence?" "Am I being overly sensitive?" In general, minority individuals are the primary people who can determine whether a comment or gesture was racially offensive to them, regardless of the offender's intentions.

Unfortunately, microaggressions can play a large role in the culturally competent care and relative comfort a minority individual may feel when seeking health care. For example, white non-Latino therapists may be unknowingly socially conditioned to hold certain cultural biases, and these may come out in their work with minority clients. While the care provider may have no intention of offending or harming their client, minority clients may feel devalued, or unheard, by white non-Latino providers who may unintentionally make racially microaggressive statements to their clients. For example, by stating to a Latino client that they need to move away from a family-centered lifestyle and focus on a more individualistic lifestyle, the therapist may be demeaning the cultural values of his or her client. Since health-care providers are typically seen as being in a position of power, minority clients may be less inclined to confront or discuss racial microaggressions uttered by their care provider. This can cause minority clients to feel less trusting toward and even cease care with their provider, which could ultimately harm the client's well-being.

Understanding and educating health-care workers about the damage created by racial microaggressions is important as they act to undervalue and minimize minority clients' efforts to articulate their needs and to comply with treatment programs. Since microaggressions are usually subtle and unintentional, educating health-care workers on what may be offensive to Mexican-origin clients as well as other minority groups is a worthwhile endeavor in supporting culturally competent care.

Understanding the Role of Gender and Cultural Competency

I'm a wife, mother, a grandmother and as you probably already know in the Latin families the mother is the pillar of the house so if I'm sick everybody's sick. The most important thing is that you keep yourself together so that your family won't fall apart, because in Latin families the mother is supposed to be the pillar so it's very hard when you're sick. I'm very lucky and blessed that my family backs me up. When I'm going downhill they'll push me back up, and that's one of the best and most important things in a Latin family is that we're tight and we're together. (Yolanda N., 52)

Yolanda's perception of gender roles is a critical component of understanding her cultural identity. In many instances both men and women project culturally appropriate behaviors in public while in private they renegotiate these roles in their daily lives. One of the major problems in training programs that focus on cultural competency is that they generalize and refer to cultural stereotypes when describing accepted gender roles.[11] Instead of conforming to a monolithic ideal of gendered behavior, it seems that most Mexican-origin women, including Mexican immigrant women, question or shift boundaries, particularly as they renegotiate their gender roles with increased acculturation, which in turn affects health behaviors.[12] Mexican-origin women define their gender roles within their culture, which will determine how receptive they may be to frank discussions on, for example, sexuality, alcohol use, or child-rearing practices. Therefore, the intersection of gender, cultural identity, and culture for Mexican American women must be understood *before* a model of culturally competent health care can be developed for these women.

Mexican immigrant and Mexican American women have largely been defined by cultural behavioral norms that describe gender relations. The terms most commonly used to describe these interactions between men and women are marianismo, **malinchismo**, machismo, and familismo. These terms, however, have also been used to describe members of the Mexican-origin population in the United States who have not assimilated into mainstream culture.

Mexican-origin and other Latina women have often been described in terms of marianismo. In *The Maria Paradox*, marianismo is defined as "the ideal role of woman . . . taking as its model of perfection the Virgin Mary herself. Marianismo is about sacred duty, self-sacrifice, and chastity. About dispensing care and pleasure, not receiving them. About living in the shadows, literally and figuratively, of your men—father, boyfriend, husband, son—your kids, and your family."[13]

Many researchers have relied on this definition without understanding the complexity of these gender stereotypes, which has resulted in a superficial description of the behavior of Mexican-origin women who reside in the United States. However, Chicana scholars view these behavioral characteristics specifically through the lens of Mexican American culture. These scholars have analyzed these behaviors in the context of the historical experiences of Mexican Americans who participated in the Chicano movement (Mexican American civil rights movement) that emerged during the 1960s. For example, citing Rendon, Angie Chabram Dernersesian explains machismo in the following manner: "The essence of machismo, of being macho, is as much a symbolic principle for the Chicano revolt as it is a guideline for family life. . . . Macho, in other words, can no longer relate merely to manhood but must relate to nationhood as well. . . . The word Chicano in many ways embodies the revolt itself."[14]

Within the context of the work of Chicana scholars, terms such as "machismo," "marianismo," and "familismo" have deeper symbolic definitions that include resistance to the dominant culture as a reaction to the historical legacy of racial discrimination in the Southwest. Moreover, Chicana feminist scholars have analyzed how Chicana/Mexican American women have resisted the negative characterization associated with ethnic and gender stereotypes. These scholars have redefined the negative connotations of many of these behavioral characteristics. This is clearly illustrated by the reconstruction of the term "malinchismo," which once symbolized the betrayal of one's culture and people, into one of resistance and strength.[15]

While gender stereotypes are sometimes reaffirmed in Mexican women's attitudes and behavior, recent works in Chicana scholarship indicate that even immigrant women question the validity of these stereotypical roles by redefining them. This literature shows a clear pattern of Mexican-origin men and women renegotiating their traditional roles as their levels of economic participation and exposure to a new social milieu alter over time. Beatríz Pesquera illustrates this pattern in her research on the division of household labor within Mexican-origin families. In Pesquera's study, traditional gender roles in Mexican-origin families were altered by the women's economic contributions to household incomes.[16]

Implementation of Cultural Competency: Implications for the Mexican-Origin Population

I think that health care providers need to start thinking outside the box, look at our communities and really go towards directing the information to where it is needed. . . . I feel that the Anglo population has a wealth of information directed to its community about exercise, about nutrition. They have exercise programs, self-help books, and so forth. They have all sorts of information, and yet that information is not reaching our communities. I don't think it is reaching the masses. . . . In terms of prevention, nutrition, diet, and the need to exercise, that message needs to be there. (Gracie S., 46)

To date there is little empirical evidence linking health-care outcomes to providers' varying levels of cultural competency. Nonetheless, the goal of cultural competency is to enhance communication skills so that individuals of different ethnic backgrounds will have greater access to cost-effective and high-quality health care, including information on preventative care. However, as illustrated previously, the theoretical and empirical base that is used for Mexican immigrants and Mexican Americans must be further developed.

The implementation of cultural competency in a health-care setting may be divided into the following three domains:

1. Acculturation models focused on developing descriptions of minority populations to assist in targeting culturally appropriate medical interventions.
2. Specific models for therapeutic treatment of identified minority groups.
3. **Process evaluation** models aimed at changing the organizational climate of the health plan or site.

These models are briefly summarized in the following sections.

Acculturation Models

I think it's important for the overall Hispanic community, whether you are Mexican, Cuban, or Puerto Rican, to learn more about the laws of the United States. And I think it is important for them to understand and get a grasp of the language. I know maybe some people don't want to learn the language, but they should at least know how to communicate with the rest of the world around them. (Martín G., 31)

Research on Latino acculturation is extensive in both the mental health and public health literatures. The importance of this research in explaining health behaviors and the health status of Latinos, particularly Mexican Americans and Mexican immigrants, cannot be overstated. For example, the acculturation scale developed by Cuellar, Harris, and Jasso is used frequently to assess the levels to which immigrant Latinos, particularly those of Mexican-origin, are acculturated into mainstream American society. Although the Cuellar scale has a number of variables related to levels of ethnic interaction as well as family and self-identification, the most significant variable is the level of English language acquisition vis-à-vis the level of native-language retention.[17] Thus, it is not surprising that level of English language proficiency becomes a critical factor in defining acculturation levels of Latinos. The pressure on immigrants who lack English proficiency to achieve economic success creates enormous psychological pressure, which can result in further isolation. According to Padilla and Salgado, "in the general literature on cross-cultural mental health, migration in and of itself is identified as a source of stress for the individual. . . . The immigrant is at high risk for experiencing severe bouts of psychosocial conflict because of self-imposed pressure to succeed and the lack of English proficiency."[18] Acculturation models predict that English language acquisition and proficiency will determine how well Latino immigrants assimilate into the dominant culture, which in turn affects their ability to access health care and health-care information.

Therapeutic Treatment Models

A large body of literature specific to therapeutic treatment can help mental health professionals assess the external issues that may be framing the behavior of minority individuals who have experienced racism. These models are not specific to the Mexican-origin population but provide some insight into the effects of discrimination on the psychosocial responses of minority clients. Thus, they provide a therapeutic framework for clinicians to treat patients suffering from depression or other psychological disorders. For example, Sue and Sue identify a common thread among all oppressed groups, which is represented in the framework of observed attitudes toward the dominant group.[19] This linear stage model uses a cultural framework to understand levels of ethnic identity formation. It enables the therapist to assess where a minority individual may "fit" within the process of identity formation. According to Sue and Sue, individuals in stage one are completely dominated by the majority group. Therefore, they exhibit a strong tendency to assimilate into the broader society and devalue their own ethnic culture relative to this dominant culture. By stage three, characteristics of resistance emerge within minority individuals, resulting in the absolute denial of the validity of the dominant culture. A self-immersion within one's ethnic culture may also occur. Finally, by stage five, the last stage, known as integrative awareness, the individual has resolved previous conflicts with the dominant society and has established his or her own identity and sense of security.[20] Cultural competency within this framework focuses on deviations from the dominant culture and identifies the extent to which a minority individual attempts to integrate into and adopt the dominant culture. These therapeutic models help to categorize observed attitudes and behaviors of minority individuals that may mediate their mental health problems.

These types of frameworks predict minority behavior in relation to the dominant culture and suggest treatment strategies based on the degree to which the individual exhibits specific levels of minority-majority integration. This model may be helpful in a clinical setting for treating specific mental health disorders. On the other hand, it may underestimate the degree to which Mexican Americans and Mexican immigrants **code switch** in both language and behavior based on a given social setting. Code switching may occur, for example, when a Mexican American patient uses idiomatic expressions and behaviors with a Mexican-origin clinician but not with a non-Mexican clinician based on an implicit assumption of cultural understanding between the two individuals. Given this implicit assumption, the patient's behavior with a non-ethnically matched health-care professional may be more guarded. In addition, the patient may attempt to adopt language and behavior that is more culturally attuned to the clinician's culture rather than relying on his or her preferred cultural behavioral norms for communication.

It is important to develop therapeutic models that consider cultural competency. However, a great deal more research is needed to assess their **efficacy in treatment** for the Mexican-origin population. A consideration of changes in cultural behavior based on the health-care environment and ethnicity of the clinician should be built into any therapeutic model used in the treatment of Mexican-origin patients.

Models of Organizational Climate

Most of the more general literature on cultural competency focuses on the organizational climate and individual behaviors of providers in specific health-care settings. Categories of acculturation may be defined with respect to language or specific cultural practices using an inventory model

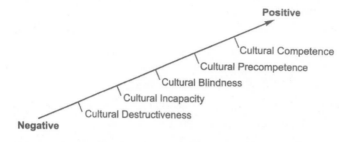

Positive

Cultural Competence
Cultural Precompetence
Cultural Blindness
Cultural Incapacity
Cultural Destructiveness

Negative

Figure 20. Continuum of cultural competence.

approach. To date, little research has focused on measuring outcomes of cultural interventions used in therapeutic treatment. Even though the body of literature on acculturation and therapeutic treatment suggests the importance of culturally competent care, there is a dearth of clinical outcome data. Nonetheless, cultural-competency training of medical staff is well underway in many health-care organizations across the country. Cultural-competency programs used for training purposes combine self-examination and criticism of provider bias using specific models that place an individual's behavior within a continuum of attitudes and behaviors (see figure 20).[21]

Assuming that a continuum of organizational behavior, ranging from culturally destructive to culturally competent, exists within health-care settings, a plan for training can be developed within these parameters. Ultimately, the goal of the multicultural or sensitivity training curriculum is for providers to become more empathetic to the needs of minority and ethnic groups by modifying the culturally destructive and culturally blind behaviors.[22]

Asking the Right Questions: Who Is a Culturally Competent Health-Care Provider?

How would you assess whether your health-care provider is culturally sensitive or culturally or linguistically competent? One way to ensure culturally and linguistically competent health care is to obtain good information about the health-care providers you are interested in or have access to. Asking friends or relatives for recommendations of Spanish-speaking or culturally sensitive health-care providers is one such strategy. Remember that it is important to ask questions regarding your health. The following are some guidelines to consider in choosing physicians, nurses, and other health-care providers who are linguistically and culturally competent:

1. Is the health-care provider of Mexican origin, Latino, or a member of another minority group?
2. Does the health-care provider share your cultural values?
3. Is the health-care provider located in your community?
4. Does the practitioner provide bilingual or interpreter services? Is the practitioner or medical staff bilingual? Can the interpreter provide adequate and accurate medical translations?
5. How well does the health-care provider listen to you? Does the person answer or dismiss your questions? Do you feel the person cares about and respects you?
6. Do you feel the health-care provider advocates for your health interests? Do you have to struggle with the practitioner when you need specialist referrals or specific medications?
7. Does the practitioner provide written materials in languages other than English?
8. Does the practitioner provide other resources and references that are linguistically and/or culturally sensitive?
9. Does the clinic provide convenient times for scheduling appointments and appointment times that accommodate your work and family schedule? Are there barriers to flexible access in terms of scheduling your medical appointments (which may include culturally or linguistically insensitive staff)?[23]

Promotores(as) de Salud: Mediators of Health

Promotores(as) de Salud, or Health Promoters (also called Community Health Workers), are representative members of underserved communities that can mediate information for health-care providers and thereby promote better health in local communities. Often, these community health leaders are used by nonprofit groups, local health clinics, and public health programs to support, educate, and increase the utilization of health-care services by community members. In general, the local knowledge promotores(as) provide at the community level allows health providers to better access these communities and provide more appropriate information to enhance compliance with regard to health screenings, preventative care, and treatment. A recent study by Reinschmidt et al. identified several characteristics of successful promotores(as): (1) a firm understanding of the community and sociocultural background of the target client group; (2) empathetic skills rooted in local knowledge that enhances perceived trust and understanding by community members; and (3) similar age match with target group and excellent bilingual, culturally competent skills, which enhance perceptions of support and caring by community members. An important outcome observed from this study was that the use of promotores(as) increased the use of preventative screenings and improved health outcomes for the targeted community members.[24]

While promotores(as) may not be health-care professionals themselves, they can play a critical role in promoting healthy communities by bridging the information gap between health-care providers and their clients. As local community members, promotores(as) understand the cultural backgrounds of their clients and can use this knowledge to help their clients access the health-care system on a more consistent basis. They can also increase their clients' opportunities to gain new knowledge about health issues at a local level that can improve their lives and those of their families.

Beyond Cultural Competency: Some Final Thoughts

> I really truly believe my doctor doesn't care about me because I'm Mexican. When I got the consultation I saw that 90 percent of his patients are Americans, white, and I'm Mexican American. I really believe that because my doctor took two months to do a blood test. It doesn't make sense. I've been calling and everything and all they say is tomorrow, tomorrow. So I really feel discriminated on that part and I don't feel good about it. (Yolanda N., 52)

A major problem that the research does not address is the underlying assumption that training medical staff in cultural competency is sufficient to enable them to provide quality health care to culturally or linguistically distinct minority groups. In general, the assumption is that any individual can be trained to become "bicompetent," that is, able to understand cultural and linguistic differences and evaluate information based on this knowledge. A fundamental problem with this assumption is that unlike language, where one can measure specific skills in spoken, written, and reading proficiency, culture is not a static domain in which one can measure specific skills. Moreover, the nature of culture as a process that individuals display when interacting with mainstream society is laden with ambiguity. As anthropologist Renato Rosaldo writes, "when in doubt, people find out about their worlds by living with ambiguity, uncertainty, or simple lack of knowledge. . . . We often improvise, learn by doing, and make things up as we go along."[25] Therefore, although certain customs and practices may indicate an individual's cultural preference, these must be interpreted with the understanding that they may not reflect key cultural factors. Some behaviors may very well be signs of hybrid biculturalism rather than reflecting a degree of acculturation within the Mexican-origin community.

Perhaps equally important in learning to become culturally competent or bicompetent is exploring oneself: one's bias, prejudices, limitations, and strengths. **Cultural humility** is a lifelong process of self-reflection and addressing those self-concepts that limit one's ability to treat others who are different with respect. Self-awareness is the key to developing respectful interactions with patients of different sociocultural backgrounds than oneself.[26]

These issues pose important questions about our ability to develop models for measuring the cultural effectiveness of health-care strategies. Given the nuances of behavior and specific cultural characteristics of the Mexican-origin population, successful health-care settings will be those that bridge the two cultures. The employment of Mexican-origin health-care professionals will be a key part of that success. Moreover, the delicate balance between ferreting out cultural-competency variables and providing a practical basis for assessing outcomes merits considerable attention and continued research. Both **process variables** and **therapeutic variables** must be clearly defined with measurable standards. However, we should be aware that how each of us defines "culture" and "language" is idiosyncratic and reflects our own life experiences. This is an important caveat for all health-care professionals because it suggests that a learned-skills approach may not be sufficient to develop a culturally competent delivery system. If it is not, then recruiting bicompetent health-care providers from specific Latino subpopulations will be necessary.

Discussion Exercises

1. Distinguish between linguistic competency and cultural competency as it relates to the health-care setting, including access to and receiving health care.

2. How would increasing the number of Mexican-origin medical staff (physicians, nurses, insurance personnel, health-care administrators) improve access to adequate and culturally competent health care?

3. What role does cultural background play in health-care issues for the Mexican-origin population?

4. How does an individual's ethnic identity (i.e., identifying as Mexican American, Chicano/a, or Latino) affect the manner in which he or she perceives the relationship with a health-care provider and health-care setting?

5. Why is it important for a clinician or health-care provider to understand the cultural differences that exist among various patients, particularly those of non-white ethnic backgrounds?

6. Distinguish between acculturation and biculturalism as it relates to the Mexican-origin population.

7. What is the biggest obstacle to implementing an optimal culturally competent health-care setting?

Notes

1. A. L. Estrada, F. M. Treviño, and L. A. Ray, "Health Care Utilization Barriers among Mexican Americans: Evidence from HHANES 1982–84," supplement, *American Journal of Public Health* 80 (1990): S30.

2. C. L. Shur and L. A. Albers, "Language, Sociodemographics, and Health Care Use of Hispanic Adults," *Journal of Health Care for the Poor and Underserved* 7, no. 2 (1996): 140–58.

3. M. Coye and D. Alvarez, *Medicaid Managed Care and Cultural Diversity in California* (San Francisco: Lewin Group, Commonwealth Fund, March 1999), v.

4. M. A. Kay, *Healing with Plants* (Tucson: University of Arizona Press, 1996), 52.

5. E. Ávila and J. Parker, *Woman Who Glows in the Dark* (New York: Jeremy P. Tarcher/Putnam, 1999); R. T. Trotter and J. A. Chavira, *Curanderismo: Mexican American Folk Healing* (Athens: University of Georgia Press, 1997).

6. California Cultural Competency Task Force, *Recommendations for the Medi-Cal Managed Care Program* (Berkeley: Institute for the Study of Social Change, University of California, Berkeley, 1994), 1.

7. D. E. Hayes Bautista, W. O. Schink, and J. Chapa, *The Burden of Support: Young Latinos in an Aging Society* (Stanford, CA: Stanford University Press, 1988), 93–114.

8. M. Raffaelli and L. L. Ontai, "'She's 16 Years Old and There's Boys Calling over to the House': An Exploratory Study of Sexual Socialization in Latino Families." *Culture, Health, & Sexuality* 3 (2001): 295–310.

9. V. L. Ruiz, "Star Struck," in *Building with Our Hands: New Directions in Chicana Studies*, ed. A. de la Torre and B. M. Pesquera, 109–29 (Berkeley: University of California Press, 1993).

10. For more information on the construction of ethnic identity by other Latino/a groups, see L. E. Guarnizo, "Los Dominicanyorks: The Making of a Binational Society," in *Challenging Fronteras: Structuring Latina and Latino Lives in the United States*, ed. M. Romero, P. Hondagneu-Sotelo, and V. Ortiz, 169–72 (New York: Routledge, 1997); J. Flores, "Qué Assimilated Brother, Yo Soy Asimilao: The Structuring of Puerto Rican Identity in the United States," in *Challenging Fronteras*, ed. Romero, Hondagneu-Sotelo, and Ortiz, 169–72; A. Portes and A. Stepick, "A Repeat Performance?: The Nicaraguan Exodus," in *Challenging Fronteras*, ed. Romero, Hondagneu-Sotelo, and Ortiz, 147; C. Nelson and M. Tienda, "The Structuring of Hispanic Ethnicity: Historical and Contemporary Perspectives," in *Challenging Fronteras*, ed. Romero, Hondagneu-Sotelo, and Ortiz, 24.

11. A. de la Torre, "Hard Choices and Changing Roles among Mexican Migrant Campesinas," in *Building with Our Hands*, ed. de la Torre and Pesquera, 168–78.

12. D. A. Segura and A. de la Torre, "La Sufrida: Contradictions of Acculturation and Gender in Latina Health," in *Revisioning Women, Health, and Healing*, ed. A. E. Clarke and V. L. Oleson, 155–63 (New York: Routledge, 1999).

13. R. M. Gil and C. I. Vazquez, *The Maria Paradox: How Latinas Can Merge Old World Traditions with New World Self-Esteem* (New York: The Berkeley Publishing Group, 1996), 7.

14. A. C. Dernersesian, "And Yes . . . The Earth Did Part," in *Building with Our Hands*, ed. de la Torre and Pesquera, 163.

15. Ibid.

16. B. Pesquera, "In the Beginning He Wouldn't Lift a Spoon: The Division of Household Labor," in *Building with Our Hands*, ed. de la Torre and Pesquera, 181–95.

17. I. Cuellar, L. C. Harris, and R. Jasso, "An Acculturation Scale for Mexican American Normal and Clinical Populations," *Hispanic Journal of Behavioral Sciences* 2, no. 3 (1980): 208.

18. A. M. Padilla and V. N. Salgado de Snyder, "Hispanics: What the Culturally Informed Evaluator Needs to Know," in *Cultural Competence for Evaluators: A Guide*

for Alcohol and Other Drug Abuse Prevention Practitioners Working with Ethnic/Racial Communities, ed. M. A. Orlandi, R. Weston, and L. G. Epstein, 117–46 (Rockville, MD: U.S. Department of Health and Human Services, Public Health Service, Alcohol, Drug Abuse, and Mental Health Administration, 1992).

19. D. W. Sue and D. Sue, *Counseling the Culturally Different* (New York: Independent Publishers Group, 1990).

20. For a more complete discussion of the model presented by Sue and Sue, see chapter 2 in P. J. Lecca et al., *Cultural Competency in Health, Social, and Human Services* (New York: Garland Publishing, 1998).

21. Lecca et al., *Cultural Competency in Health, Social, and Human Services*, 51–54.

22. Ibid., 52–54.

23. For more information on cultural competency, see Arizona Hispanic Center of Excellence, University of Arizona website: http://hispanichealth.arizona.edu/; or The National Conference of State Legislatures Resources for Cross-Cultural Health Care Henry J. Kaiser Family Foundation, Diversity Rx website: www.diversity Rx.org.

24. K. M. Reinschmidt et al., "Understanding the Success of Promotoras in Increasing Chronic Diseases Screening," *Journal of Health Care for the Poor and Underserved* 17, no. 2 (May 2006): 256–64.

25. R. Rosaldo, *Culture and Truth: The Remaking of Social Analysis* (Boston: Beacon Press, 1989), 152.

26. L. M. Hunt, "Beyond Cultural Competence: Applying Humility to Clinical Settings," in *The Social Medicine Reader*, 2nd ed., vol. 2, ed. N. M. P. King, R. P. Strauss, L. R. Churchill, S. E. Estroff, G. E. Henderson, and J. Oberlander (Durham, NC: Duke University Press, 2005).

Suggested Readings

Ávila, E., and J. Parker. *Woman Who Glows in the Dark*. New York: Jeremy P. Tarcher/ Putnam, 1999.

Cross, T., B. Bazron, E. Dennis, and M. Isaacs. *Toward a Culturally Competent System of Care*. Vol. 1. Washington, DC: CASSP, Georgetown University, 1989.

Dean, R. G. "Understanding Health Beliefs and Behaviors: Some Theoretical Principles of Practice." In *Removing Cultural and Ethnic Barriers to Health Care*, ed. E. L. Watkins and A. E. Johnson, 49–67. Chapel Hill: University of North Carolina Press, 1979.

Desmond, J. "Communicating with Multicultural Patients." *Life in Medicine* (1994): 7–25.

Harwood, A. *Ethnicity and Medical Care*. Cambridge, MA: Harvard University Press, 1981.

Isaacs, M. R., and M. P. Benjamin. "Toward a Culturally Competent System of Care: A Monograph on Effective Services for Minority Children Who Are Severely Emotionally Disturbed." In *Monographs of Programs Which Utilize Culturally Competent Principles*, Vol. 2. Washington, DC: CASSP, Georgetown University, 1991.

Kay, M. *Healing with Plants.* Tucson: University of Arizona Press, 1996.

————. *Spanish-English, English-Spanish Medical Dictionary of the Southwest.* 2nd ed. Tucson: University of Arizona Press, 2001.

Lecca, P. L., I. Quervalú, J. V. Nunes, and H. F. Gonzales. *Cultural Competency in Health, Social, and Human Services.* New York and London: Garland Publishing, 1998.

Office of Minority Health Resource Center website, Cultural Competency Resources: http://www.asianhealthservices.org/.

Pernell-Arnold, A. *Diversity and Health Care Training.* (Training curricula). Philadelphia: APAC, 1995.

Power, J. G., and T. Byrd. *U.S.-Mexico Border Health: Issues for Regional and Migrant Populations.* Thousand Oaks, CA: Sage Publications, 1998.

Pulido, L. *Environmentalism and Economic Justice: Two Chicano Struggles in the Southwest.* Tucson: University of Arizona Press, 1996.

Trotter, R. T., II, and J. A. Chavira, *Curanderismo: Mexican American Folk Healing.* 2nd ed. Athens: University of Georgia Press, 1997.

U.S. Department of Health and Human Services. Surgeon General's National Hispanic/Latino Health Initiatives. *One Voice, One Vision—Recommendations to the Surgeon General to Improve Hispanic/Latino Health.* Washington, DC: Government Printing Office, 1993.

Chapter 6

Future Trends in Mexican American Health

"This Is about Healing, about People Getting Better Prevention"

There are many important issues to consider in assessing the health of the Mexican-origin population in the United States. The health of this group influences the overall data on Latino health, as Mexican-origin people make up the largest Latino subpopulation. Even though data are often combined under the broad category "Latino or Hispanic," it is necessary to differentiate between subgroups. For this reason, we have sought to outline key factors that influence the health status and access issues of Mexican Americans wherever possible. With the rapid growth of the Latino population, it is becoming increasingly important to have research that provides information specific to Latino subgroups. Such information is necessary to the development of more effective health interventions and policies.

As indicated at the beginning of the text, we focus on the geographic concentration of Mexican Americans in the Southwest as well as their long-time presence in this region, which predates the United States Declaration of Independence. Their large presence in the border region has had a direct impact on the health risk factors they experience. Mexican Americans' historical experience as a colonized people since the United States' annexation of the Southwest has played an important role in their current social status. Their present-day experiences in schools and the labor market are to a significant degree the result of the history of the American Southwest. This history, in which language issues and racial and ethnic discrimination figure prominently, has had a large impact on the general health of Mexican Americans.[1]

Health does not exist in isolation from historical, socioeconomic, or cultural factors. For example, cultural values, beliefs, and attitudes influence health-seeking behaviors. Cultural values such as familismo, personalismo, confianza, dignidad, and respeto affect the patient-provider relationship and may influence health-care outcomes. It is, therefore, important to understand Mexican Americans' level of acculturation in relation to their health because the strength of these cultural values will vary with acculturation level. Many of the diseases that we have reviewed are influenced by the Mexican American cultural environment. Acknowledging cultural issues, therefore, is an essential part of any prevention and treatment program.

When we look at the health status of Mexican Americans by age, we find that children suffer from problems such as underimmunization, obesity, and periodontal disease. Adolescents suffer from increasing rates of Type II diabetes and from high mortality rates due to motor vehicle accidents, homicides, and suicides. Mexican American adolescents also tend to begin sexual activity early, which increases other health risks including unintended pregnancies and HPV infection. Adults also suffer from Type II diabetes, which is correlated with metabolic syndrome and obesity, among other factors. Late diagnosis and poor medical management of Type II diabetes in the adult population create additional problems such as peripheral vascular disease. This in turn can lead to the amputation of limbs and to blindness. Heart disease is the leading cause of death among all racial and ethnic groups in the United States, and cancer is the second leading cause of death among Latinos. The three most common forms of cancer among Mexican-origin men are lung cancer, colorectal cancer, and prostate cancer. For Mexican-origin women, breast cancer, lung cancer, and colorectal cancer are most common. A lack of knowledge about and access to screenings for these cancers in many cases gets in the way of early diagnosis and effective treatment.

Acquired immunodeficiency syndrome is the fourth leading cause of death among Latinos. However, the epidemiology of HIV disease is different for Mexican Americans than for other groups. For example, a large number of Mexican-born men contract the virus through male-male sex, whereas Mexican-born women acquire the virus primarily through sex with an HIV-positive male. Only a small percentage of Mexican-born women acquire HIV through injection drug use. Unfortunately, there are a number of misconceptions among Mexican Americans concerning HIV transmission, and improved outreach and education are needed in this community. Other areas of concern that directly affect the health status of Mexican Americans are prenatal care, IPV, occupationally related health diseases, and communicable and parasitic diseases related to low-income housing and occupational location.

With the complete mapping of the human genome in the early twenty-first century, it is now possible to examine specific genes and their contribution to the etiology of disease in human populations. Recent research has examined the specific contribution of Native American ancestry and disease risk among Mexican-origin Latinos, among others. These studies have found a significant association between the proportion of Native American admixture and diseases such as Type II diabetes, obesity, asthma, cardiovascular disease, and breast cancer.[2] The importance of these discoveries lies in the development of early genetic screening and the implementation of gene-therapy to treat these diseases.[3]

Health-care access is a significant problem for all Mexican Americans. Access refers not only to financial access (i.e., health insurance) but also to issues such as the proximity of medical facilities and the availability of culturally and linguistically appropriate care. With the recent passage of the Affordable Care Act (ACA) under the Obama administration, we can feel optimistic that access to affordable health insurance will increase the number of insured in the United States. Nevertheless, the Mexican-origin population constitutes an exceptionally large percentage of this uninsured population, and the challenges of integrating them into this new health financing system are multiple. Factors influencing health insurance coverage include not only occupational location and economic status but also the ineligibility of many Mexican-origin people for publicly subsidized health insurance due to their immigrant status. Undocumented immigrants are the most vulnerable of this group.

A final important component of health-care access concerns the availability of minority health-care professionals: doctors, nurses, psychologists, and others. The scarcity of Mexican-origin health-care professionals diminishes the quality of health care for Mexican Americans, who are already underserved. Mexican-origin health-care professionals play an important role because they are more likely to serve in their respective communities and to bridge the gap between the culture of this minority group and that of the health-care system. Therefore, increasing the number of Mexican-origin health-care professionals will enable more Mexican Americans to access care. Medical school educational pipeline programs such as PRIME at the University of California are important models for increasing the number of health-care professionals in underserved Mexican-origin communities.

Another important factor that influences access to quality health care is the degree of cultural and linguistic competency of the professionals serving people of Mexican descent. Linguistic competency is important to many Mexican immigrants. Monolingual Spanish speakers are at particular risk of not receiving adequate health care. It is well known that Spanish-speakers with limited English proficiency (LEP) tend to receive less information about therapeutic regimens, understand less of the instructions related to their medication, are less likely to make follow-up visits, and are less likely to receive preventative care. Thus, linguistic competency is an essential component of cultural competency.

Cultural competency requires that individuals who serve the Mexican-origin population understand and be sensitive to the values, practices, and beliefs of this group. Effective communication is a critical component of cultural competency. Cultural competency includes not only the language the population uses but also sensitivity to the literacy levels of this group and how their cultural and belief systems inform their health-care practices. Of equal importance is the practice of self-reflection and self-awareness on the part of the health professional as a means of embracing cultural humility. More research is needed on how to create effective programs that assist health professionals in attaining cultural competence, especially with Mexican-origin populations.

The models that are most frequently used in understanding cultural competency in the health-care setting fall into three frameworks: acculturation, therapeutic treatment, and organizational process. Each of these models has some limitations with respect to its application to Mexican-origin people. For example, the spectrum of ethnic identity within the Mexican-origin population tends to be reduced to the single issue of linguistic skills in Spanish and in English. Given the increasingly complex identity of the Mexican-origin population—which includes such factors as immigration status, generational status, and regional location—cultural-competency models must become more sensitive to the unique characteristics of specific Mexican-origin communities. For example, the cultural identity of Mexicans who live in the border regions of Texas or Arizona may be closer to that of Mexican nationals than, say, to that of **Hispanos/ as** of northern New Mexico. Thus, some cultural and linguistic practices differ substantially.

Cultural competency requires that we look at the mix of our health-care providers as well as the support given to individuals who enter the health-care system. Individuals who are trained to be culturally competent may still lack an intuitive understanding of the culture. Thus, it is important that we continually strive to increase the pool of Mexican-origin health-care professionals as well as improve the skills of existing practitioners.

What needs to be done to improve the health status of Mexican Americans in the twenty-first century? A number of Latino health providers and researchers (including the authors of this book) examined this issue in collaboration with the Surgeon General of the United States as early as 1993.[4] With the exception of the emerging measures for health-care reform under the PPACA of 2010, the following areas were identified in the Surgeon General's report as needing improvement:

1. Access to health care
2. Data collection strategies
3. Representation in the sciences and health professions
4. Development of a relevant and comprehensive research agenda
5. Culturally appropriate health promotion and disease prevention programs

Areas in need of improvement with regard to health-care access include:

1. Comprehensive and portable health-care coverage. PPACA will tackle this issue, but major barriers remain for undocumented immigrants.
2. Latinos in leadership positions affecting public policy.
3. Adequate and available health-care service delivery systems and infrastructure to address primary, secondary, and tertiary health-care needs of Latinos.
4. Accessible and adequate health-care facilities to address financial, cultural, and linguistic barriers.

Problems identified in the area of data collection include:

1. Inadequate inclusion of Latinos in data systems
2. Lack of data specific to Latino health issues
3. Limited awareness of and access to local, state, and federal databases
4. Lack of quality, accurate, timely, and culturally sensitive data system design, collection efforts, analysis, and replication

5. Poor coordination of efforts in health data collection by local, state, and federal agencies

Problems identified with respect to representation in the health professions include:

1. The underrepresentation of Latinos at all levels of the health professions
2. The underrepresentation of Latinos in the educational pipeline of the health professions, as well as inadequate levels of funding for Latinos in health and science education programs
3. The underutilization of linguistically and culturally competent foreign-educated Latino health professionals

Problems identified in the area of research agendas include:

1. Underfunding of Latino health research initiatives
2. Lack of culturally appropriate theories, models, and methodologies
3. Underrepresentation of Latinos at all levels of research activities
4. Lack of coordination among diverse areas of investigation

Problems identified in the area of health promotion and disease prevention include:

1. Weak infrastructure for training in health promotion and disease prevention
2. Lack of proven models for comprehensive, culturally competent, and community-specific primary, secondary, and tertiary prevention programs
3. Lack of public-private partnerships in support of health promotion and disease prevention goals
4. Lack of diffusion of culturally appropriate health promotion and disease prevention models
5. General lack of awareness on the part of media and the public about Latino health promotion and disease prevention issues
6. Lack of cooperation in addressing environmental hazards that affect health promotion and disease prevention

Over the last twenty years progress has been made in some of these areas. This progress can be partially explained by the demographic growth of this population, which has resulted in greater political engagement and the growing political clout of the Mexican-origin and Latino communities in the Southwest and nationally. Latinos, who experienced a 43 percent increase in population between 2000 and 2010 and are one of the fastest growing populations in the United States, have attracted attention both in terms of their economic and political clout. Latinos are also a young population; just under four million Latinos reached the voting age between 2008 and 2012. These demographic trends have allowed Latinos to increase their voter mobilization in several key elections. Latinos made up 8.4 percent of the voters in the 2012 election (up 1 percent from the 2008 presidential election). Latinos' political engagement in these areas is important; President Obama's success in the 2012 election was due to the strong Latino vote he received in vital swing states. Nevertheless, despite these important gains, only a few national and regional Latino advocacy groups promote the types of issues outlined above. Key groups advocating for important policy changes with regard to Latino health include: The National Hispanic Medical Association, the National Council of La Raza, the National Immigration Law Center, the Latino Coalition for a Healthy California, and regional foundations such as the California Endowment. These groups have made a concerted effort to involve local, state, and national health policymakers in collaborations with Latino health professionals and the community at large to address many of the issues presented by the Surgeon General's report and have improved health access for this growing community. The future of the United States depends on a healthy, educated, and motivated citizenry. Given the Mexican-origin and Latino community's increasing political empowerment and the growing sophistication of their advocacy groups and community leaders, the next decade should create the right opportunities for reducing disparities in health care and status. By highlighting the issues that need to be addressed if Mexican-origin people are to overcome the obstacles they have faced in the past and by suggesting interventions and strategies for doing so, this text serves as a roadmap by which they can continue to make important improvements in their health into the twenty-first century.

Concluding Thoughts

This text has highlighted several important health issues affecting the Mexican-origin population in the United States as well as strategies for improvement. As of this writing little progress has been achieved in implementing immigration reform for the estimated eleven million undocumented persons living in the United States. This lack of progress raises concerns that the problem of inadequate access to health care for this population will remain an unresolved problem, particularly in states such as Arizona and Texas where undocumented immigrants have limited financial access through publicly subsidized health-care systems. At the same time, the PPACA enrolled over eight million people in its first year, surpassing the Congressional Budget Office's initial projection of seven million; just over half of those individuals enrolled in federally facilitated exchanges.[5] These numbers bode well for the success of this program despite the broader congressional and state-level political bickering over its implementation and the differential access to care across state boundaries. Moreover, even though the training of health professionals in cultural competency has become a major concern in the delivery of health care to Latinos, few studies have evaluated the efficacy of this approach in reducing health disparities among this population or increasing the number of culturally competent health-care professionals. The nation's future is in many ways dependent on the younger, immigrant population for its economic strength and political stability. As such, sustained and aggressive efforts to increase the health of the Mexican-origin population should be at the forefront of health policy issues for the twenty-first century.

Discussion Exercises

1. What is the association between Native American ancestry and health status among Mexican-origin Latinos?

2. What issues did the Surgeon General identify as priorities in 1993?

3. Why is it important to reduce health disparities among Mexican-origin populations residing in the United States?

4. Which Latino cultural values are associated with health outcomes?

5. What is known about the efficacy of cultural competency in the delivery of health care?

6. How do federal policies impact access to care for the Mexican-origin population, and which policies must be reformed if we are to create greater social equity within the Mexican-origin population?

Notes ·

1. A. L. Estrada, "Mexican Americans and Historical Trauma Theory: A Theoretical Perspective," *Journal of Ethnicity in Substance Abuse* 8, no. 3 (2009): 330–40.

2. J. M. Galanter et al., "Cosmopolitan and Ethnic-Specific Replication of Genetic Risk Factors for Asthma in 2 Latino Populations." *Journal of Allergy and Clinical Immunology* 128 (2011): 37–43.e12; H. Wu et al., "Evaluation of Candidate Genes in a Genome-Wide Association Study of Childhood Asthma in Prevalence and Type of *BRCA* Mutations in Hispanics Undergoing Genetic Cancer Risk Assessment in the Southwestern United States: A Report from the Clinical Cancer Genetics Community Research Network," *Journal of Allergy and Clinical Immunology* 125 (2010): 321–7.e13; J. N. Weitzel et al., "Prevalence and Type of *BRCA* Mutations in Hispanics Undergoing Genetic Cancer Risk Assessment in the Southwestern United States: A Report from the Clinical Cancer Genetics Community Research Network," *Journal of Clinical Oncology* 31 (2012): 210–16; V. Acuna-Alonzo et al., "A Functional ABCA1 Gene Variant Is Associated with Low HDL-Cholesterol Levels and Shows Evidence of Positive Selection in Native Americans," *Human Molecular Genetics* 19, no. 14 (2010): 2877–85; V. L. Martinez-Marignac et al., "Admixture in Mexico City: Implications for Admixture Mapping of Type 2 Diabetes Genetic Risk Factors," *Human Genetics* 120 (2007): 807–19; J. R. Fernandez and M. D. Shriver, "Using Genetic Admixture to Study the Biology of Obesity Traits and to Map Genes in Admixed Populations," *Nutrition Reviews* 62, no. 7 (July 2004): S69–S74.

3. A. Moreno-Estrada, C. R. Gignoux, J. C. Fernández-López, et al., "The Genetics of Mexico Recapitulates Native American Substructure and Affects Biomedical Traits," *Science* 344 (2014): 1280; N. A. Johnson et al., "Ancestral Components of Admixed Genomes in a Mexican Cohort," *PLOS Genetics* 7, no. 12 (2011): e1002410 [doi:10.1371/journal.pgen.1002410]; R. Voelker, "Promising Test Flags *BRCA* Mutations in Populations of Hispanic Women," *Journal of the American Medical Association* 301, no. 13 (April 1, 2009): 1326–27.

4. A. Novello, *Recommendations to the Surgeon General to Improve Hispanic/Latino Health* (Washington, DC.: U.S. Department of Health and Human Services, Office of the Surgeon General, June 1993).

5. H. Adamopoulos, 6 Key Statistics on PPACA Enrollment for 2014, *Becker's Hospital Review* (May 1, 2014), retrieved from http://www.beckershospitalreview.com/.

Suggested Readings

Bustamante, A. V., J. Chen, H. P. Rodriguez, J. A. Rizzo, and A. N. Ortega. "Use of Preventive Care Services among Latino Subgroups." *American Journal of Preventive Medicine* 38, no. 6 (2010): 610–19.

Daviglus, M. L., G. A. Talavera, M. L. Avilés-Santa, M. Allison, J. Cai, M. H. Criqui, M. Gellman, A. L. Giachello, N. Gouskova, R. C. Kaplan, L. LaVange, F. Penedo, K. Perreira, A. Pirzada, N. Schneiderman, S. Wassertheil-Smoller, P. D. Sorlie, and J. Satmler. "Prevalence of Major Cardiovascular Risk Factors and Cardiovascular Diseases among Hispanic/Latino Individuals of Diverse Backgrounds in the United States." *Journal of the American Medical Association* 308, no. 17 (2012): 1775–84.

Gonzalez, H. M., W. A. Vega, and W. Tarraf. "Health Care Quality Perceptions among Foreign-Born Latinos and the Importance of Speaking the Same Language." *Journal of the American Board of Family Medicine* 23, no. 6 (November–December 2010): 745–52.

National Healthcare Disparities Report 2012. DHHS, Agency for Healthcare Research and Quality, AHRQ Publication No. 13–0003, May 2013: www.ahrq.gov/.

GLOSSARY

acculturation   The degree to which *Mexican Americans* adopt mainstream, Euro-American values and customs. It usually refers to the learning of two cultures—Mexican American and Euro-American.

acculturative stress   Psychosocial stress associated with the process of modifying one's culture through contact with another culture group (*acculturation*) or of adapting to the dominant culture.

AIDS (acquired immunodeficiency syndrome)   Disease of the human immune system that is caused by infection with HIV.

allopathic   Describes an approach to medicine that views the physician as an active interventionist. A physician who practices this type of medicine attempts to counteract the effect of a disease by using surgical or medical treatments that produce effects opposite to those of the disease.

American Association of Medical Colleges   An organization of *allopathic* colleges of medicine in the United States and Canada.

Arizona's HB 2281   A house bill passed in 2010 by the Arizona state legislature. It was broadly interpreted in Arizona as a ban on ethnic studies programs such as the Mexican-American Studies program housed within the Tucson Unified School District. The bill included the following elements: classes must not promote resentment toward an ethnic group, must not be designed for the pupils of a particular ethnic group, and must not advocate ethnic solidarity.

attributable risk   The rate of disease that can be directly linked to exposure to a disease.

backloading   A means of sharing drugs by squirting part of the drug solution into the back of the syringe.

behavioral epidemiology   A specialty in the field of epidemiology; it focuses on risk behaviors that contribute to the spread of disease.

bicultural   Having the ability to operate in two cultures. This requires skill in the language, knowledge of cultural norms, and the ability to switch between the expectations of two distinct cultures.

bilingual   Having or using two languages. The fluency of a native speaker is implied in the definition.

bilis   A hot, dry condition resulting from bile secretion that is emitted when an individual is suffering from chronic rage.

birth rate   The number of live births per 1,000 women in a population.

Chicano/Chicana People of Mexican American descent who have re-evaluated how their ethnic awareness affects the way they see themselves within the Mexican American and broader communities.

code switch The ability to shift between two languages or dialects based on the ethnic makeup of a specific group in order to appropriately match the expected communication style of that group.

confianza A sense of confidence or trust in one's health-care provider or physician; the establishment of a trusting, safe, and open bond between two people.

co-occurrence Things that happen together or simultaneously.

cooker A spoon, bottle cap, or concave part of an aluminum can that is used to heat, dissolve, and rinse a drug solution.

cotton Fabric used to filter a solution of drugs before injection.

cultural competency The acceptance and respect for cultural differences. To be culturally competent, medical staff must self-assess their attitudes and agency policies regarding culture, must pay careful attention to the dynamics of difference, must continually expand their cultural knowledge and resources, and must change their service models in order to better meet the needs of the client population.

cultural humility Self-reflection and self-evaluation of one's own bias, prejudices, and beliefs in order to become more respectful in interactions with people from different cultural backgrounds.

curandera/curandero A folk healer whose practice of healing is based on the use of native plants and herbs in curative potions and the laying on of the hands. This method of healing is widespread in Latin America, the Caribbean, and the southwestern United States.

de facto segregation Segregation that is actual but not necessarily supported or enforceable by law or legislation.

de jure segregation Segregation that is supported or enforceable by law, legislation, or administrative policies.

dignidad A Mexican American/Chicano's personal sense of dignity.

educational attainment The highest grade completed or the highest educational degree obtained by an individual. The average education level of a population group can be calculated using these data.

educational pipeline An academic path to a career that requires higher education. To increase the number of minorities in a field, the educational pipeline ideally would have primary and secondary schools with high graduation rates for under-represented minority (URM) students, colleges interested in increasing the number of URM graduates going on to medical school or postgraduate study in health sciences, and "academic medical centers" (medical schools and other health professional schools) that want to improve opportunities for URM students and health-care professionals.

efficacy in treatment The ability or power to give cost-effective treatment that results in the best possible health outcomes.

empacho A swollen belly resulting from undigested food.

epidemiological Of or relating to *epidemiology*, which is the study of disease patterns and distributions in human groups.

epidemiological patterns Risk factors, risk behaviors, *incidence* rates, and *prevalence* rates of disease.

epidemiological profile A complete picture of how a population group is affected by disease. It is based on a combination of risk factors, risk behaviors, *incidence* rates, and *prevalence* rates.

epidemiology The study of disease patterns and distributions in human populations.

ethnic enclaves Migrants or *immigrants* of a similar background or from the same region that reside close together. Generally, enclaves are sites of mutual assistance, where residents share resources and information with each other.

etiology All of the causes of a disease or condition.

familismo The cultural belief that places family needs above individual needs and desires.

federal poverty level (FPL) The guideline for determining poverty in the United States. In the forty-eight states and Washington, DC, a family of four is considered to live in poverty if their annual income is at or below the federal poverty line of $23,850.

feminization of poverty A term that describes the increasing numbers of single-parent households where women are the head of the household. An overly large number of these women and their children are living in poverty.

fertility rate The number of live births per 1,000 women between the ages of fifteen and forty-four in a specified population group.

financial access The ability either to pay for private health insurance or to qualify for free or low-cost public health-care coverage.

foreign-born All U.S. residents who were not born either in the United States or in a U.S. territory or to a parent who is a U.S. citizen.

frío de la matriz This term literally translates as "cold womb or cold uterus." It is a folk disease that is recognized after a mother has given birth (postpartum). It is believed to be caused by insufficient rest after delivery. Symptoms include pelvic congestion, menstrual irregularities, and loss of libido.

frontloading The process of drawing a drug solution from a *cotton* or *cooker* through the needle of a syringe.

Gadsden Purchase A piece of land that the United States bought from Mexico for $10 million in 1853. It is named after Senator James Gadsden, who negotiated the sale. Measuring about 30,000 square miles, it includes what is today southern New Mexico and southern Arizona.

Grutter v. Bollinger A court case in which the Supreme Court ruled that affirmative-action programs could be in place if the racial status of a college applicant was one factor used to determine enrollment eligibility in the interest of maintaining diversity within the student body.

health-care access The opportunity to obtain and pay for health-care services and procedures. Access is often affected by income, employment, and language status.

health insurance premium The price of insurance protection for a specified risk for a specified period of time. Many health insurance plans require payment of monthly premiums.

health status A measure of an individual's or a population's health based on many psychological and physical factors, such as mortality and morbidity rates (number of deaths and number of people with diseases that may cause death). Health status varies greatly among different ethnic groups and is related to income, *educational attainment*, and race/ethnicity.

healthy migrant hypothesis The idea that migrants from Mexico are generally healthier than other American minority populations. This hypothesis attempts to explain the Mexican American mortality-morbidity paradox (that is, the fact that *Mexican Americans* have lower rates of death and serious illness than do other minority groups).

Hippocratic-Galenic beliefs Beliefs that come from Greek humoral theory (proposed by Hippocrates) and expanded upon by Galen (a Roman physician). This theory says that there are four humors, or fluids, in the body: black bile, yellow bile, blood, and phlegm. An imbalance in these four humors was believed to cause certain illnesses.

Hispanic   Of, relating to, or being a person of Latin American descent living in the United States. Included are people of Cuban, Mexican, Puerto Rican, Central American, or South American origin.

Hispano/Hispana   A native or resident of the U.S. Southwest who is a descendant of Spaniards who settled in the area before it was taken over by the United States. It is most often used to refer to long-time *Hispanic* residents of New Mexico.

HIV (human immunodeficiency virus)   One of a group of viruses called retroviruses. HIV gradually destroys certain white blood cells called T-helper lymphocytes. The result is that the body cannot control viruses or bacteria that the normal immune system keeps in check easily. *AIDS* (*acquired immunodeficiency syndrome*) refers to the disease process caused by HIV infection.

home health agency   A business that arranges for health-care professionals to examine and treat patients in their own homes.

Hopwood decision   The 1996 ruling that the affirmative action admissions policy of the University of Texas law school had resulted in discrimination against four white applicants. This decision resulted in the removal of all affirmative action programs in Texas institutions of higher education as illegal. "Race neutral" policies were put in place to determine admission, financial aid, scholarships, recruitment, and retention programs.

immigrants   A category of *foreign-born* people who come to the United States from another country to live for an indefinite period of time; not all *foreign-born* persons are immigrants.

incidence   The number of new cases of an illness or disease that occurs in a certain population at a particular time. It measures how many people are currently becoming infected or affected by a disease and is one measure of morbidity.

inpatient care   Health-care procedures that require the patient to stay in the hospital for a time. It is the opposite of outpatient treatment.

la sufrida   The "suffering" woman; la sufrida is based on the concept of *marianismo*, a Mexican/Chicano/*Latino* cultural expectation that women should be self-sacrificing.

Latino/Latina   A person who is a native or inhabitant of Western Hemisphere countries that are south of the United States, including

Mexico, Central and South America, and the Caribbean; it also applies to a person living in the United States who comes, or whose ancestors come, from one of these countries.

linguistic competency   The ability to speak, read, and write the language of a specific population and also to understand the nuances of the region, class position, and preferred dialect of the specific group.

longitudinal data   Data that are collected over a long period of time. The same measures are collected on the same individuals at set intervals over a span of years. Longitudinal data allow one to understand how a problem develops and progresses.

machismo   Manliness and virility. The lighter side of machismo within *Latino* cultures is personified by the *caballero* (gentleman) who is responsible for the welfare of his family and protects the honor of his wife and family. It is also associated with a man's sexual prowess with women. Machismo is expressed in romanticism as a jealous guarding of one's wife or fiancé and as premarital and extramarital affairs.

mal de ojo   An illness caused by being stared at; usually perceived in children or babies who have been paid more attention than usual; the illness also has a supernatural component.

malinchismo   A concept that embodies the historical role of Malinche or Doña Marina, the Aztec princess who served as Cortés' interpreter, guide, and mistress during the conquest of Mexico. It can be used as a negative term describing Mexican-origin women who are seen as traitors against Mexican culture or the Mexican-origin community.

marianismo   The female counterpart of *machismo*. Taken from the name Mary, it is based on the figure of the Virgin Mother within the Catholic religion. For example, women are expected to suffer in silence with regard to the sexual double standard and their husband's affairs, to place their children's and husband's needs above their own, and to be the overseer of the home and family (including health-care issues).

matriculants   Applicants to a medical or other school who have been accepted to the school and have chosen to enroll there.

Medicaid   A jointly funded, federal-state health insurance program for low-income and needy people. Coverage includes children, people who are elderly, blind, or disabled, and people who are eligible for federal income maintenance payments (welfare, SSI). More recently Medicaid expansion has been included as an additional health insurance option within several state ACA insurance exchanges.

medically indigent   Describes a person who is too poor to pay for medical care and does not have private or public health insurance. State medically indigent programs may provide both cash and medical assistance, or medical assistance only.

Medicare   This Federal program provides health insurance to people age sixty-five and over, those with permanent kidney failure, and certain people with disabilities. To be eligible for Medicare, an individual or his or her spouse must have worked for at least ten years in Medicare-covered employment, be at least sixty-five years of age, and be a citizen or permanent resident of the United States.

metropolitan area   A geographic area of large population. It includes a core city (or cities) and nearby communities that are socially and economically connected to it. For example, a metropolitan area could be composed of an urbanized city and the communities from which the city's workers commute.

Mexican American mortality-morbidity paradox   This is based on empirical observations that *Mexican Americans*, due to protective cultural factors, have lower rates of death and serious illness than do other minority groups.

Mexican Americans   Persons of Mexican descent born and residing in the United States.

modifiable risk factors   Health behaviors that put a person at risk for illness but that can be adjusted or changed to lower the risk. Examples are lifestyle choices such as smoking, lack of exercise, and poor diet.

morbidity   The number of people in a population at any given time who have a particular disease, illness, or injury; the rate of *incidence* of a disease.

mortality   The number of deaths in a population for a given period of time.

native-born   A U.S. resident born within the United States or in a U.S. territory (for example, Puerto Rico), or born in a foreign country to an American citizen.

natural history of disease   The natural cycle of a disease, which includes the growth of or infection with a disease resulting in illness, death, or recovery.

non-insulin-dependent diabetes mellitus (NIDDM)   The most common form of diabetes mellitus; about 90 to 95 percent of people who have diabetes have NIDDM, also called Type II diabetes. Unlike the insulin-dependent type of diabetes (Type I), in which the pancreas makes no insulin, people with non-insulin-dependent diabetes produce some insulin, sometimes even large amounts. However, either their bodies do not produce enough insulin or their body cells do not take in insulin properly. People with NIDDM can often control their condition through diet, exercise, and weight loss.

non-Latino   People who do not identify themselves as Mexican American, Chicano/a, Mexican, Mexicano/a, Puerto Rican, Cuban, Central American, South American, or other *Hispanic*.

obesity   The state of being significantly overweight. Anyone who is more than 20 percent over his or her ideal weight is considered obese.

occupational location   The type of job and sector of employment (e.g., manufacturing, service) in which a person is employed.

outpatient health services   Health-care procedures that can be done without an overnight stay in a hospital.

Pap smear   A test for cancer in the female genital tract in which a small sample of cells is scraped off the cervix for testing.

partera   Midwife.

patchwork providers   A loose association of health-care providers that provide health-care services for the underinsured or uninsured in a given region.

personalismo   The capacity to appreciate and build on personal relationships to establish meaningful bonds of communication and trust. Personalismo is a cultural attribute that builds on the importance of extended kinship relationships in Mexican culture.

predictor variables   The influencing factors used to forecast or identify a particular relationship between the past and future occurrence of a behavior or to determine a pattern of behavior.

prevalence   The number of people in a certain population at a certain time who have a given disease or injury; the "measurement of *morbidity* at a point in time." Whereas *incidence* measures only new cases of a disease or illness, prevalence measures all the people affected by that condition, no matter how long they have had it.

primary prevention Efforts to stop a disease before it occurs. Behavioral modification tools that are important in primary prevention include health promotion, health education, and health protection.

process evaluation Assessments obtained during health promotion activities that are used to control, provide feedback on, or improve the quality of performance or delivery of the program.

process variable The adaptation of organizational systems and the development of health professional interpersonal skills that support cultural elements that enhance communication between the patient and the health care provider.

Proposition 209 A 1996 initiative to do away with affirmative-action programs and policies in all state and local governments, districts, public universities, colleges, schools, and other government agencies in the state of California.

psychologically inoculate To provide resistance skills that lower the risk for using drugs.

racialized A situation in which groups are defined or categorized based on biological identifying characteristics.

razalogía The empowerment of *raza* communities (Chicana/o/Latino/a). A primary goal of this empowerment is to support protective cultural behaviors that strengthen the overall community's well-being through each member's strong cultural/ethnic identification.

relative risk The risk of disease or death in a population exposed to a health condition divided by the risk of disease or death in the unexposed population.

respeto Mutual respect between physician and patient that should be maintained; demonstrates professionalism and understanding of boundaries in the relationship; the need to maintain one's personal integrity and that of others.

rinse water Water that is used to flush out or rinse a syringe before or after use.

salmon bias hypothesis The idea that Mexican-origin persons return to Mexico to die, preventing them from being recorded in death statistics.

SCHIP State Children's Health Insurance Program; implemented in the late 1990s to help provide health insurance to low-income families with children.

secondary prevention   Efforts to screen for or detect a disease or illness in an early stage to prevent it from progressing to an impairment or disability.

seroprevalence   A measure of the *prevalence* or extent of the HIV virus in the blood of a particular population.

simpatía   A state in which social interactions are smooth and positive.

sobadora   A healer who practices massage therapy using spiritual or religious principles.

speedball   An injected mixture of heroin and cocaine.

subjective culture   The non-physical aspects of a culture, including attitudes, norms, values, beliefs, and expectancies.

subpopulation   An identifiable section or subdivision of a population.

Supplemental Security Income (SSI)   A federal program that provides income to people who are sixty-five or older, blind, or disabled and who have few assets or little income. Children are included.

susto   Fright of the soul; the perceived loss of one's soul due to a frightening or traumatic event that creates an imbalance.

syncretism   The mixture or combination of different cultural or religious forms of belief, practice, or ritual.

syndemic   The coming together of several *epidemics* such as substance abuse, *HIV/AIDS*, and violence.

tertiary prevention   Efforts designed to slow or stop the progression of a disability, condition, or disorder to minimize the amount of care required.

therapeutic variable   The integration of elements of a patient's culture into specific interventions used by health professionals in the treatment of a mental, physical, or spiritual illness.

Treaty of Guadalupe Hidalgo   The peace treaty that ended the Mexican War on February 2, 1848, signed in the town of Guadalupe Hidalgo outside Mexico City. It granted Texas to the United States and officially set the U.S.-Mexico border at the Rio Grande. Mexico also ceded California and the land that would become the states of Nevada and Utah, as well as parts of present-day Arizona, New Mexico, Colorado, and Wyoming. The United States paid Mexico $15 million for this territory. The treaty also promised that Mexicans living in the territory ceded to the United States would receive full rights as U.S. citizens.

variable In scientific research, a measurable element or factor that does or might influence an outcome or situation. For example, variables influencing *health status* include *occupational location*, socioeconomic status, immigrant status, and *educational attainment*.

voluntary system of health insurance A system that deducts an amount from an individual's paycheck and allows the person to pay into a private health insurance plan instead of being forced to participate in the program provided by the employer.

working poor Individuals who are active in the labor force but do not receive fringe benefits such as health insurance.

BIBLIOGRAPHY

Abraido-Lanza, A. F., B. P. Dohrenwend, D. S. Ng-Mak, and J. B. Turner. "The Latino Mortality Paradox: A Test of the 'Salmon Bias' and Healthy Migrant Hypotheses." *American Journal of Public Health* 89 (1999): 1543–48.

Aizcorbe, A., E. Liebman, S. Pack, D. M. Cutler, M. E. Chernew, and A. B. Rosen. "Measuring Health Care Costs of Individuals with Employer-Sponsored Health Insurance in the U.S.: A Comparison of Survey and Claims Data." *Statistical Journal of the IAOS* 28 (1/2): 43–51.

Al-Samarrai T., A. Madsen, R. Zimmerman, G. Maduro, W. Li, C. Greene, and E. Begier. "Impact of a Hospital-Level Intervention to Reduce Heart Disease Overreporting on Leading Causes of Death." *Preventing Chronic Disease* 10 (2013): 120–210. DOI: http://dx.doi.org/.

Alfaro, P. "Horizontes Laredo Indigenous Outreach Project." In *Community-Based AIDS Prevention*, 15–17. DHHS Pub. No. (ADM) 91–7752. Washington, DC: U.S. Department of Health and Human Services, 1991.

Alvarez, R. *Latino Community Mental Health.* Spanish Speaking Mental Health Research and Development Program Monograph No. 1. Los Angeles: University of California at Los Angeles, 1974.

American Cancer Society. Cancer Facts and Figures for Hispanics/Latinos 2012–2014. Atlanta, GA: American Cancer Society, 2012. Website: http://www.cancer.org/.

———. Cancer Facts and Figures 2010. Atlanta, GA: American Cancer Society, 2010. Website: http://www.cancer.org/.

American Community Survey. S2701: "Health Insurance Coverage Status." In *2009 American Community Survey 1-Year Estimates.*

———. S0201: "Selected Population Profile in the United States." In *2009 American Community Survey 1-Year Estimates.*

American Diabetes Association. *Diabetes Statistics.* Retrieved on November 5, 2010, from http://www.diabetes.org/.

American Heart Association. "Overweight and Obesity: Statistics." Statistical Fact Sheet: Risk Factors, 2009. Retrieved on November 9, 2010, from http://www.americanheart.org/.

American Lung Association. "Lung Cancer Fact Sheet." Retrieved August 22, 2013, from http://www.lung.org/.American Nurses Association website: http://www.ana.org/.

Andrade, S. J., and C. Doria-Ortiz. "Nuestro Bienestar: A Mexican-American Community-Based Definition of Health Promotion in the Southwestern United States." *Drugs: Education, Prevention, and Policy* 2, no. 2 (1995): 129–45.

Angel, J. L, J. K. Montez, and R. J. Angel. "A Window of Vulnerability: Health Insurance Coverage among Women 55 to 64 Years of Age." *Women's Health Issues* (2010): available online at http://www.utexas.edu/.

Arizona Health Care Cost Containment System website: http://www.azahcccs.gov/.

Association of American Medical Colleges website: http://www.aamc.org/.

Association of American Medical Colleges. *Diversity in Medical Education: Facts and Figures 2008.* Washington, DC: Association of American Medical Colleges, 2008.

———. *Facts: Applicants, Matriculants, and Graduates, 1991–1997.* U.S. 1997/1998 ed. Washington, DC: Association of American Medical Colleges, 1998.

———. *Project 3000 by 2000 Progress to Date: Year Four Progress Report.* Washington, DC: Association of American Medical Colleges, Division of Community and Minority Programs, 1996.

Ávila, E., and J. Parker. *Woman Who Glows in the Dark.* New York: Jeremy P. Tarcher/Putnam, 1999.

Barrera, M. *Race and Class in the Southwest: A Theory of Racial Inequality.* Notre Dame, IN: University of Notre Dame Press, 1979.

Barzansky, B., H. S. Jonas, and S. I. Etzel. "Education Programs in U.S. Medical Schools, 1997–1998." *Journal of the American Medical Association* 280 (1998): 803–8.

Bayer, R. "AIDS Prevention and Cultural Sensitivity: Are They Compatible?" *American Journal of Public Health* 84 (1994): 895–98.

Bolen, J. C., L. Rhodes, E. E. Powell-Griner, S. D. Bland, and D. Holtzman. "State-Specific Prevalence of Selected Health Behaviors, by Race and Ethnicity: Behavioral Risk Factor Surveillance System, 1997." *Mortality and Morbidity Weekly Report* 49 (SS02) (March 24, 2000): 1–60.

Booth, R. E., J. K. Watters, and D. D. Chitwood. "HIV Risk-Related Sex Behaviors among Injection Drug Users, Crack Smokers, and Injection Drug Users Who Smoke Crack." *American Journal of Public Health* 83, no. 8 (1993): 1144–48.

Botvin, G. J., S. P. Schinke, J. A. Epstein, and T. Diaz. "The Effectiveness of Culturally Focused and Generic Skills Training Approaches to Alcohol and Drug Abuse Prevention among Minority Youth." *Psychology of Addictive Behaviors* 8 (1994): 116–27.

Boyko, E. J., E. M. Keane, J. A. Marshall, and R. F. Hamman. "Higher Insulin and C-peptide Concentrations in Hispanic Populations at High Risk for NIDDM: San Luis Valley Diabetes Study." *Diabetes* 40 (1991): 509–15.

California Attorney General's Office website: http://Vote96.ss.ca.gov/.

California Secretary of State's Office website: http://ca94.election.digital.com/.

Campbell, K. M. "The Road to S.B. 1070: How Arizona Became Ground Zero for the Immigrants' Rights Movement and the Continuing Struggle for Latino Civil Rights in America." *Harvard Latino Law Review* 14: 1–21.

Casas, J. M. "A Culturally Sensitive Model for Evaluating Alcohol and Other Drug Abuse Prevention Programs: A Hispanic Perspective." In *Cultural Competence for Evaluators: A Guide for Alcohol and Other Drug Abuse Prevention Practitioners Working with Ethnic/Racial Communities*, ed. M. A. Orlandi, R. Weston, and L. G. Epstein, 75–116. Rockville, MD: U.S. Department of Health and Human

Services, Public Health Service, Alcohol, Drug Abuse, and Mental Health Administration, 1992.

Centers for Disease Control and Prevention (CDC). *The Health of America's Youth: Current Trends in Health Status and Health Services.* Atlanta, GA: CDC, 1991.

————. Cancer Prevention and Control. "Cancer among Men." Retrieved March 2013 from http://www.cdc.gov/.

————. Cancer Prevention and Control. "Cancer among Women." Retrieved January 2013 from http://www.cdc.gov/.

————. *Diabetes Data and Trends: Diagnosed Diabetes by Race/Ethnicity, Age and Sex.* Retrieved on November 5, 2010, from http://www.cdc.gov/.

————. Division for Heart Disease and Stroke Prevention. "Women and Heart Disease Fact Sheet." Retrieved August 22, 2013, from http://www.cdc.gov/.

————. "Diagnoses of HIV Infection and AIDS in the United States and Dependent Areas 2008." June 14, 2010–November 9, 2010. Available at: http://www.cdc.gov/.

————. "Differences in Prevalence of Obesity among Black, White, and Hispanic Adults: United States, 2006–2008," *Mortality and Morbidity Weekly Report* (July 17, 2009).

————. "Drug Use and Sexual Behaviors among Sex Partners of Injecting-Drug Users: United States, 1988–1990." MMWR. *Morbidity and Mortality Weekly Report* 40, no. 49 (1991): 855."What Is Medicare?" June 4, 1999. Available at: http://www.medicare.gov/.

————. "High Blood Pressure." February 1, 2010–June 22, 2010. Available at: http://www.cdc.gov/.

————. *HIV/AIDS Surveillance Report.* Year-end edition. Vol. 10, no. 2. Washington, DC: U.S. Department of Health and Human Services, Public Health Service, 1998.

————. "HIV Surveillance in Injection Drug Users." Retrieved July 10, 2011, http://www.cdc.gov/.

————. "HIV/AIDS among Hispanics/Latinos." October 8, 2009–November 9, 2010. Available at: http://www.cdc.gov/.

————. *National Diabetes Fact Sheet: National Estimates and General Information on Diabetes and Prediabetes in the United States, 2011.* Atlanta, GA: U.S. Department of Health and Human Services, Centers for Disease Control and Prevention, 2011. Available at: http://www.cdc.gov/.

————. *National Diabetes Surveillance System.* Retrieved on November 6, 2010, from http://apps.nccd.cdc.gov/.

————. *NCHS Health E-Stat, Prevalence of Obesity among Children and Adolescents: United States Trends, 1963–1965 Through 2007–2008.* Retrieved November 4, 2010, from http://www.cdc.gov/.

————. *Office of Minority Health and Health Disparities: 10 Leading Causes of Death Hispanic/Latino Population, 2006.* Retrieved on November 8, 2010, from http://www.cdc.gov/.

———. "Self-Reported Prevalence of Diabetes among Hispanics: United States, 1994–1997." *Mortality and Morbidity Weekly Report* 48, no. 1 (1999): 8–12.

———. *Suicide: Facts at a Glance*. Retrieved on November 5, 2010, from http://www.cdc.gov/.

———. *The Burden of Oral Disease: Tool for Creating State Documents*. Atlanta: U.S. Department of Health and Human Services, 2005. Available at: http://www.cdc.gov/.

———. *Vaccines and Immunizations, Statistics and Surveillance: 2009 Table Data*. Retrieved November 4, 2010, from http://www.cdc.gov/.

———. *Vaccines and Immunizations, Statistics and Surveillance: July 2008–June 2009 Table Data*, retrieved November 4, 2010, from http://www.cdc.gov/.

———. Youth Risk Behavior Surveillance—United States, 2009. Surveillance Summaries, June 4, 2010. *Morbidity and Mortality Weekly Report* 59, no. SS-5 (2010): 1–148.

———. Cancer Prevention and Control. "Rates of New Lung Cancer Cases." November 23, 2009–November 8, 2010. Available at: http://www.cdc.gov/.

Center for Substance Abuse Prevention. *Advanced Methodological Issues in Culturally Competent Evaluation for Substance Abuse Prevention*. Health Resources and Services Administration Bureau of Primary Health Care. Rockville, MD: U.S. Department of Health and Human Services, 1996.

Chabram-Dernersesian, A., and A. de la Torre. "A Retrospective on the Narratives of Latina Health: What We Can Learn." In *Speaking From the Body: Latinas on Health and Culture*, ed. A. Chabram-Dernersesian and A. de la Torre, 154–72. Tucson: University of Arizona Press, 2008.

Chávez, E. L., F. Beauvais, and E. R. Oetting. "Drug Use by Small-Town Mexican American Youth: A Pilot Study." *Hispanic Journal of Behavioral Science* 8, no. 3 (1986): 243–58.

Chávez, E. L., R. Edwards, and E. R. Oetting. "Mexican American and White American Dropouts' Drug Use, Health Status, and Involvement in Violence." *Public Health Reports* 104, no. 6 (1986): 594–604.

Chávez, E. L., and R. C. Swain. "An Epidemiological Comparison of Mexican American and White Non-Hispanic 8th and 12th Grade Students' Substance Use." *American Journal of Public Health* 82 (1992): 445–47.

Cohen, J. B., L. B. Hauer, and C. B. Wofsy. "Women and IV Drugs: Parental and Heterosexual Transmission of Human Immunodeficiency Virus." *Journal of Drug Issues* 19, no. 1 (1989): 39–56.

Cohen, L. M. "*Controlarse* and the Problems of Life among Latino Immigrants." In *Stress and Hispanic Mental Health: Relating Research to Service Delivery*, 202–18. DHHS Pub. No. (ADM) 85–141. Washington, DC: U.S. Department of Health and Human Services, 1985.

Collins, K. S., D. L. Hughes, M. M. Doty, B. L. Ives, J. N. Edwards, and K. Tenney. "Diverse Communities, Common Concerns: Assessing Health Care Quality for Minority Americans, Findings from the Commonwealth Fund 2001 Health Care Quality Survey." *Commonwealth Fund*, 2002, 1–68. Retrieved on November 3, 2010, from http://www.commonwealthfund.org/.

Colorado Department of Health Care Policy and Financing website: www.chcpf. state.co.us/.

The Columbia Encyclopedia, 5th ed. New York: Columbia University Press, n.d. Accessed at CBS News website: http://cbs.infoplease.com/.

COSSMHO (National Coalition of Hispanic Health and Human Service Organizations) *HIV/AIDS—The Impact on Hispanics in Selected States*. Washington, DC: COSSMHO, 1991.

Cuellar, I., B. Arnold, and R. Maldonado. "Acculturation Rating Scale for Mexican Americans–II: A Revision of the Original ARSMA Scale." *Hispanic Journal of Behavioral Sciences* 17, no. 3 (1995): 275-304.

Daviglus, M. L, G. A. Talavera, M. L. Avilés-Santa, M. Allison, J. Cai, M. H. Criqui, M. Gellman, A. L. Giachello, R. Gouskova, R. C. Kaplan, L. LaVange, F. Penedo, K. Perreira, A. Pirzada, N. Schneiderman, S. Wassertheil-Smoller, P. D. Sorlie, and J. Stamler. "Prevalence of Major Cardiovascular Risk Factors and Cardiovascular Diseases among Hispanic/Latino Individuals of Diverse Backgrounds in the United States." *Journal of the American Medical Association* 308, no. 17 (2012): 1775–84.

Dávila, A., A. K. Bohara, and R. Saenz. "Accent Penalties and the Earnings of Mexican Americans." *Social Science Quarterly* 74, no. 4 (December 1993): 902–16.

Davis, S. M., and M. B. Harris. "Sexual Knowledge, Sexual Interests, and Sources of Sexual Information of Rural and Urban Adolescents from Three Cultures." *Adolescence* 17, no. 66 (1982): 471–92.

Dawson, D. A., and A. M. Hardy. "AIDS Knowledge and Attitudes among Hispanic Americans: Provisional Data from the 1988 National Health Interview Survey." *NCHS Advance Data* 166 (1990): 1–22.

De Anda, D., R. M. Becerra, and P. Fielder. "Sexuality, Pregnancy, and Motherhood among Mexican American Adolescents." *Journal of Adolescent Research* 3 (1988): 403–11.

de la Torre, A. "Hard Choices and Changing Roles among Mexican Migrant Campesinas." In *Building with Our Hands: New Directions in Chicana Studies*, ed. A. de la Torre and B. M. Pesquera, 168–78. Berkeley: University of California Press, 1993.

de la Torre, A., R. Friis, H. R. Hunter, and L. García. "The Health Insurance Status of U.S. Latino Women: A Profile from the 1982–1984 HHANES." *American Journal of Public Health* 86, no. 4 (April 1996): 533–37.

De la Trinidad, M. "Mexican Americans in Education: Segregation in the Southwest Schools, 1930–1976." Unpublished seminar paper, Department of History, University of Arizona, 1998.

Dembo, R., J. Schmeidler, C. C. Sue, P. Borden, D. Manning, and M. Rollie. "Psychosocial, Substance Abuse, and Delinquency Differences among Anglo, Hispanic, and African American Male Youths Entering a Juvenile Assessment Center." *Substance Use and Misuse* 33, no. 7 (1998): 1481–1510.

Department of Health and Human Services website: http://aspe.os.dhhs.gov/.

Department of Health and Human Services, Health Insurance Marketplace: Summary Enrollment Report for the Period: October 1, 2013–February 19, 2014, ASPE Issue Brief, May 1, 2014.

Des Jarlais, D. C., M. E. Chamberland, S. R. Yancovitz, P. Weinberg, and S. R. Friedman. "Heterosexual Partners: A Large Risk Group for AIDS [letter]." *Lance* 2, no. 8415 (1984): 1346–47.

Díaz, T., J. W. Buehler, K. G. Castro, and J. W. Ward. "AIDS Trends among Hispanics in the United States." *American Journal of Public Health* 83 (1993): 504-509.

DiClemente, R. J., C. B. Boyer, and E. S. Morales. "Minorities and AIDS: Knowledge, Attitudes and Misconceptions among Black and Hispanic Adolescents." *American Journal of Public Health* 78, no. 1 (1988): 55–57.

Dye, B. A., S. Tan, V. Smith, B. G. Lewis, L. K. Barker, and G. Thornton-Evans. "Trends in Oral Health Status: United States, 1988–1994 and 1999–2004: National Center for Health Statistics." *Vital and Health Statistics* 11, no. 248 (2007): 1–104.

"Eliminating Racial and Ethnic Disparities in Health." Washington, DC: Grant Makers in Health, September 1998.

Ennis, S. R., M. Rios-Vargas, and N. G. Albert. "The Hispanic Population: 2010." *2010 Census Briefs*, U.S. Department of Commerce, Economics and Statistics Administration, United States Census Bureau.

Espinosa, K. E., and D. S. Massey. "Determinants of English Proficiency among Mexican Migrants to the United States." *International Migration Review* 31, no. 1 (Spring 1997): 28–50.

Espinosa, P. "The Border" (series broadcast on PBS). Available at: www.pbs.org/.

Espinoza L., H. I. Hall, R. M. Selik, and X. Hu. "Characteristics of HIV Infection among Hispanics, United States 2003–2006." *Journal of Acquired Immune Deficiency Syndrome* 49 (2008): 94–101.

Estrada, A. L. "Behavioral Epidemiology of HIV Risks among Injection Drug Users: Comparative Assessment." Paper presented at the HIV-AIDS Health Services Research and Delivery Conference, Agency for Health Care Policy and Research, Miami, Fla., December 1991.

———. "Deriving Culturally Competent HIV Prevention Models for Mexican American Injection Drug Users." In *National Institute on Drug Abuse Conference*,

AIDS Prevention Intervention among Minority Injecting Drug Users: Collected Papers. Washington, DC: U.S. Department of Health and Human Services, April 1992.

———. "Drug Use and HIV Risks among African-American, Mexican-American, and Puerto Rican Drug Injectors." *Journal of Psychoactive Drugs* 30, no. 3 (1998): 247–53.

———. "HIV Risk Behaviors among Gay Latinos Residing in the U.S.-Mexico Border Area." Paper presented at the 120th Annual Meeting of the American Public Health Association, Washington, DC, April 1992.

———. "Epidemiology of HIV/AIDS, Hepatitis B, Hepatitis C, and Tuberculosis among Minority Injecting Drug Users." Supplement, *Public Health Reports* 117 (2002): S126–S34.

Estrada, A. L., J. R. Erickson, S. J. Stevens, and P. J. Glider. "AIDS Risk Behaviors among Straight and Gay IVDUS: A Comparative Analysis." Paper presented at the Second Annual National AIDS Demonstration and Research NADR Conference, Bethesda, MD, November 1990.

———. "HIV Risk Behaviors among Mexican-Origin and Anglo Female Intravenous Drug Users." *Border Health* 7, no. 1 (1991): 1–4.

"Excerpts from Don and Mike's Messages of Hatred to Hispanics," *Hispanic Link Weekly Report* 17, no. 34 (August 30, 1999).

Flack, J. M., H. Amaro, W. Jenkins, S. Kunitz, J. Levy, M. Mixon, and E. Yu. "Epidemiology of Minority Health." *Health Psychology* 14, no. 7 (1995): 592–600.

Flora, J. A., and C. E. Thoresen. "Reducing the Risk of AIDS in Adolescents." *American Psychologist* 43, no. 11 (1988): 965–70.

Freire, P. *Pedagogy of the Oppressed.* New York: Continuum, 1995.

Friedman-Jiménez, G., and J. S. Ortiz. "Occupational Health." Chapter 12 in *Latino Health in the United States: A Growing Challenge*, ed. C. W. Molina and M. Aguirre-Molina. Washington, DC: American Public Health Association, 1994.

Fryar, C. D., T. Chen, and X. Li. Prevalence of Uncontrolled Risk Factors for Cardiovascular Disease: United States, 1999–2010. NCHS data brief, no. 103. Hyattsville, MD: National Center for Health Statistics, 2012.

Gavin, N. I., E. K. Adams, K. E. Hartmann, M. B. Benedict, and M. Chireau. "Racial and Ethnic Disparities in the Use of Pregnancy-Related Health Care among Medicaid Pregnant Women." *Maternal and Child Health Journal* 8 (2004): 113–26.

Gavira, M., and G. Stem. "Problems in Designing and Implementing Culturally Relevant Mental Health Services for Latinos in the United States." *Social Science Medicine* 14B (1980): 65–71.

Gergen, P. J., T. Ezzati, and H. Russell. "DTP Immunization Status and Tetanus Antitoxin Status of Mexican American Children Ages Six Months through Eleven Years." *American Journal of Public Health* 78 (1988): 1446–50.

Giachello, A. "Maternal/Perinatal Health." Chapter 6 in *Latino Health in the United States: A Growing Challenge*, ed. C. W. Molina and M. Aguirre-Molina. Washington, DC: American Health Association, 1994.

Gil, R. M., and C. I. Vázquez. *The Maria Paradox: How Latinas Can Merge Old World Traditions with New World Self-Esteem*. New York: Perigee Books, 1996.

Ginzburg, H. M. "Intravenous Drug Users and the Acquired Immune Deficiency Syndrome." *Public Health Reports* 99 (1984): 206–12.

Glaser, N. S., and K. L. Jones. "Non-insulin Dependent Diabetes Mellitus in Mexican American Children." *Western Journal of Medicine* 168, no. 1 (1998): 11–16.

Grant, B. F., F. S. Stinson, D. S. Hasin, D. A. Dawson, P. Chou, and K. Anderson. "Immigration and Lifetime Prevalence of DSM-IV Psychiatric Disorders among Mexican Americans and Non-Hispanic Whites in the United States." *Archives of General Psychiatry* 61 (2004): 1226–33.

Gray, L. "S.C. Has Fastest Growing Hispanic Population in the Nation." *Spartanburg Herald Journal*, 2008. Retrieved October 2, 2010, from http://www.goupstate.com/.

Gutiérrez, D. G. *Walls and Mirrors*. Berkeley: University of California Press, 1995.

Guyer, J., and C. Mann. "Employed but Not Insured: A State-by-State Analysis of the Number of Low-Income Working Parents Who Lack Health Insurance." Washington, DC: Center on Budget and Policy Priorities, 1999. Available at: http://www.cbpp.org/.

Haffner, S. M., M. P. Stern, H. P. Hazuda, M. Rosenthal, J. A. Knapp, and R. M. Malina. "Role of Obesity and Fat Distribution in Non-insulin Dependent Diabetes Mellitus in Mexican Americans and Non-Hispanic Whites." *Diabetes Care* 9 (1986): 153–61.

Hamamoto, D. Y., and R. Torres. *New American Destinies: A Reader in Contemporary Asian and Latino Immigration*. New York: Routledge, 1997.

Harris, M., K. M. Flegal, C. C. Cowie, M. S. Eberhardt, D. E. Goldstein, R. R. Little, H. M. Wiedmeyer, and D. D. Byrd-Holt. "Prevalence of Diabetes, Impaired Fasting Glucose, and Impaired Glucose Tolerance in U.S. Adults: The Third National Health and Nutrition Examination Survey, 1988–1994." *Diabetes Care* 21 (1998): 518–24.

Health Care Financing Administration website: http://www.hcfa.gov/.

Health Care Financing Administration. "Medicaid." Available at: http:www.hcfa.gov/.

Health Resources and Services Administration, Division of Disadvantaged Assistance, Centers of Excellence website: http://www.hrsa.dhhs.gov/.

Herbst, J. H., L. S. Kay, W. F. Passin, C. M. Lyles, N. Crepaz, and B. V. Marín, for the HIV/AIDS Prevention Research Synthesis (PRS) Team. "A Systematic Review and Meta-Analysis of Behavioral Interventions to Reduce HIV Risk Behaviors of Hispanics in the United States and Puerto Rico." *AIDS and Behavior* 11 (2007):

25–47, HIV/AIDS Prevention Research Synthesis Project, retrieved on July 11, 2011, from http://www.CDC.gov/.

Heron, M. National Vital Statistics Reports, *Deaths: Leading Causes for 2006* 58, no. 14 (2010): 1–100.

Hidalgo, M. "Language and Ethnicity in the 'Taboo' Region: The U.S.-Mexico Border." *International Journal of Sociology of Language* 114 (1995): 29–45.

Hingson, R., L. Strunin, D. E. Craven, L. Mofenson, T. Mangione, B. Berlin, H. Amaro, G. A. Lamb. "Survey of AIDS Knowledge and Behavior Changes among Massachusetts Adults." *Preventive Medicine* 18 (1989): 806–16.

Hoefer, M., N. Rytina, and B. C. Baker. "Estimates of the Unauthorized Immigrant Population Residing in the United States: March 2012." *Office of Immigration Statistics, Population Estimates Homeland Security* (2012): 1–7. Ibañez, G. E., D. W. Purcell, R. Stall, J. T. Parsons, and C. A. Gómez. "Sexual Risk, Substance Abuse, and Psychological Distress in HIV-Positive Gay and Bisexual Men Who also Inject Drugs." Supplement, *AIDS* 19, no. S1 (2005): S49–S55.

Immigration and Naturalization Service. "Illegal Alien Resident Population." Available at: http://www.ins.usdoj.gov/.

Impact Consultants. School-Based Survey Report for 6th and 10th Graders in Yuma County, Arizona, 1995. Tucson, AR: Impact Consultants.

Instituto Nacional de Estadística, Geografía, e Informática website: www.inegi.gob .mx/economia/espanol/feconomia.html.

Ismail, A. I., and S. M. Szpunar. "The Prevalence of Total Tooth Loss, Dental Caries, and Periodontal Disease among Mexican Americans, Cuban Americans, and Puerto Ricans: Findings from HHANES 1982–1984." Supplement, *American Journal of Public Health* 80 (1990): S66–S70.

Johnson-Kozlow, M., S. Roussos, L. Rovniak, and M. Hovell. "Colorectal Cancer Test Use among Californians of Mexican Origin: Influence of Language Barriers." *Ethnicity and Disease* 19 (2009): 315–22.

Johnston, L. D., P. M. O'Malley, and J. G. Bachman. The Monitoring the Future Study, 1975–1998, vol. 1. Washington, DC: U.S. Department of Health and Human Services, 1999.

Johnston, L. D., P. M. O'Malley, J. G. Bachman, and J. E. Schulenberg. Demographic Subgroup Trends for Various Licit and Illicit Drugs, 1975–2010 (Monitoring the Future Occasional Paper No. 74). Ann Arbor, MI: Institute for Social Research. Available at: http://www.monitoringthefuture.org/

Jórquez, J. S. "The Retirement Phase of a Heroin Using Career." *Journal of Drug Issues* 13 (1983): 343–65.

Kass, B. L., R. M. Weinick, and A. C. Monheit. "Racial and Ethnic Differences in Health 1996." MEPS Chartbook No. 2. Available at Agency for Health Care Policy Research website: www.meps.ahcpr.gov/papers/chartbk2/chartbk2a.htm.

Kegeles, S. M., N. E. Adler, and C. E. Irwin Jr. "Sexually Active Adolescents and Condoms: Changes over One Year in Knowledge, Attitudes, and Use." *American Journal of Public Health* 78 (1988): 460–61.

Klevens, J. "An Overview of Intimate Partner Violence among Latinos." *Violence Against Women* 13, no. 2 (February 2007): 111–22.

Klor de Alva, J. J. "The Invention of Ethnic Origins and the Negotiation of Latino Identity, 1969–1981." In *Challenging Fronteras: Structuring Latina and Latino Lives in the United States*, ed. M. Romero, P. Hondagneu-Sotelo, and V. Ortiz, 55–71. New York: Routledge, 1997.

Lecca, P. J., I. Quervalú, J. V. Nunes, and H. F. Gonzales. *Cultural Competency in Health, Social, and Human Services: Directions for the Twenty-First Century*. New York: Garland Publishing, 1998.

Lloyd-Jones, D., R. Adams, M. Carnethon, G. De Simone, T. B. Ferguson, K. Flegal, E. Ford, K. Furie, A. Go, K. Greenlund, N. Haase, S. Hailpern, M. Ho, V. Howard, B. Kissela, S. Kittner, D. Lackland, L. Lisabeth, A. Marelli, M. McDermott, J. Meigs, D. Mozaffarian, G. Nichol, C. O'Donnell, V. Roger, W. Rosamond, R. Sacco, P. Sorlie, R. Stafford, J. Steinberger, T. Thom, S. Wasserthiel-Smoller, N. Wong, J. Wylie-Rosset, and Y. Hong, for the American Heart Association Statistics Committee and Stroke Statistics Subcommittee. (2009). Heart Disease and Stroke Statistics: 2009. Update: A Report from the American Heart Association Statistics Committee and Stroke Statistics Subcommittee. *AHA Statistical Update*, American Heart Association.

MacMillan, M. "Evaluation and Treatment of Patients from Nonwhite Ethnic Groups." Paper presented at the 132nd annual meeting of the American Psychiatric Association, Chicago, 1979.

Manoleas, P., ed. *The Cross-Cultural Practice of Clinical Case Management in Mental Health*. New York: Haworth Press, 1996.

Marin, G. "AIDS Prevention among Hispanics: Needs, Risk Behaviors, and Cultural Values." *Public Health Reports* 104 (1989): 411–15.

———. "Defining Culturally Appropriate Community Interventions: Hispanics as a Case Study." *Journal of Community Psychology* 21 (1993): 149–61.

Markides, K. S., D. J. Lee, and L. A. Ray. "Acculturation and Hypertension in Mexican Americans." *Ethnicity and Disease* 3, no. 1 (1993): 70-74.

Martin, J. A., B. E. Hamilton, P. D. Sutton, S. J. Ventura, F. Menacker, S. Kirmeyer, and M. L. Munson. "Births: Final Data for 2005." National Vital Statistics Reports 56, no. 6. Hyattsville, MD: National Center for Health Statistics, 2007.

Martinez, A. N., R. N. Bluthenthal, N. M. Flynn, R. L. Anderson, and A. H. Kral. "HIV Risks and Seroprevalence among Mexican American Injection Drug Users in California." *AIDS Behavior*, Online First (2009).

Martinez, G. (2010). "Learning from Proposition 187: California's Past Is Arizona's Prologue." Retrieved August 22, 2013, from http://www.americanprogress.org/.

Martínez, O. J. *Border People: Life and Society in the U.S.-Mexico Borderlands*. Tucson: University of Arizona Press, 1994.

Mata, A. *Alcohol Use among Rural South Texas Youth*. Austin: Texas Commission on Alcohol and Drug Abuse, 1986.

Medicare website: http://www.medicare.gov/.

MedicineNet online medical dictionary: www.medicinenet.com.

Mexperience. "Mexico in Facts and Figures." January 2010. Retrieved on November 21, 2010, from http://www.mexperience.com/.

Milliman and Robertson Actuaries and Consultants website: http://www.blueworld .com/.

Miranda, M. R., ed. *Psychotherapy with the Spanish-Speaking: Issues in Research and Service Delivery*. Spanish Speaking Mental Health Research Center Monograph No. 3. Los Angeles: University of California at Los Angeles, 1976.

MMWR, *Drug Induced Deaths—United States, 2003–2007*, January 14, 2011/60(01):60–61, retrieved July 12, 2011, from http://www.cdc.gov/.

Modern Language Association (MLA). *Statement on Tucson Mexican American Studies Program*. Retrieved on November 13, 2014, from http://www.mla.org/.

Montoya, I. D., A. L. Estrada, A. Jones, and R. R. Robles. "An Analysis of Differential Factors Affecting Risk Behaviors among Out-of-Treatment Drug Users in Four Cities." *Drugs and Society* 9 (1996): 155–71.

Moore, D. S., and P. I. Erickson. "Age, Gender, and Ethnic Differences in Sexual and Contraceptive Knowledge, Attitudes, and Behaviors." *Family and Community Health* 8 (1985): 38–51.

Morse, A., P. Mbachu, and A. Hermes. "2012 immigration-Related Laws, Bills and Resolutions in the States: Jan.1-March 31, 2012." Retrieved August 22, 2013, from http://www.ncsl.org/.

Mosher, W. D., and J. W. McNally. "Contraceptive Use at First Premarital Intercourse: United States, 1965–1988." *Family Planning Perspectives* 23 (1991): 108–16.

Myers, M. H., F. Snyder, E. Bryant, and P. Young. "Report on Reliability of the AIDS Initial Assessment Questionnaire." In *Community-Based AIDS Prevention*. DHHS Pub. No. (ADM) 91–1752, pp. 167–82. Washington, DC: U.S. Department of Health and Human Services, 1991.

National Adolescent Health Information Center, *National Data Project: Homicide Mortality*, retrieved November 28, 2010, from http://nahic.ucsf.edu/.

National Cancer Institute (2013). "Cancer Statistics Fast Stats." Retrieved August 22, 2013, from http://seer.cancer.gov/.

National Center for Health Statistics. *Deaths of Hispanic Origin: Vital and Health Statistics* ser. 20, no. 18 (1990).

———. *Health, United States, 1998 (with Socioeconomic Status and Health Chartbook)*. Hyattsville, MD: U.S. Department of Health and Human Services, 1998.

————. *Health, United States, 1993.* Available at: http://www.cdc.gov/.

————. *Health, United States, 2009: With Special Feature on Medical Technology.* Hyattsville, MD: U.S. Department of Health and Human Services, 2010.

————. *Health, United States, 2009*, table 141. Hyattsville, MD: U.S. Department of Health and Human Services, 2010.

National Institute on Drug Abuse. *National Household Survey on Drug Abuse: Population Estimates 1991.* DHHS Pub. No. (ADM) 92–1887. Washington, DC: U.S. Department of Health and Human Services, 1991.

————. 2003. *Drug Use among Racial/Ethnic Minorities* (NIH Publication No. 03–3888). Bethesda, MD. Retrieved on November 15, 2010, from http://archives .drugabuse.gov/.

————. "Use of Selected Drugs among Hispanics: Mexican-Americans, Puerto Ricans, and Cuban Americans." Findings from the Hispanic Health and Nutrition Examination Survey. Washington, DC: U.S. Department of Health and Human Services, 1987.

National Institutes of Health website: www.niddk.nih.gov/health/diabetes/pubs /dmdict/dmdict.htm.

National Institutes of Health. *Drug Use among Racial/Ethnic Minorities.* NIH Pub. No. 98–3888. Bethesda, MD: National Institutes of Health, 1998.

————. *Morbidity and Mortality: 2009 Chart Book on Cardiovascular, Lung, and Blood Diseases*, Retrieved on November 8, 2010, from http://www.nhlbi.nih.gov/.

————. "Study First to Show Mexican Americans Hospitalized More Often for Heart Attack than Non-Hispanic Whites." NIH Pub. #97–4517. Bethesda, MD: National Institutes of Health, 1997.

Negy, C., and D. J. Woods. "The Importance of Acculturation in Understanding Research with Hispanic Americans." *Hispanic Journal of Behavioral Sciences* 14, no. 2 (1992): 224–47.

Nelson, C., and M. Tienda. "The Structuring of Hispanic Ethnicity: Historical and Contemporary Perspectives." In *Challenging Fronteras: Structuring Latina and Latino Lives in the United States*, ed. M. Romero, P. Hondagneu-Sotelo, and V. Ortiz, 7–27. New York: Routledge, 1997.

Neufeld, D., L. J. Raffel, C. Landon, Y. D Chen, and C. M. Vadheim. "Early Presentation of Type 2 Diabetes in Mexican American Youth." *Diabetes Care* 21 (1998): 80–86.

Norris, A. E., and K. Ford. "Condom Beliefs in Urban, Low Income, African American and Hispanic Youth," *Health Education and Behavior* 21, no. 1 (1994): 39–53.

Novello, A. *Recommendations to the Surgeon General to Improve Hispanic/Latino Health.* Washington, DC: U.S. Department of Health and Human Services, Office of the Surgeon General, June 1993.

The Office of Minority Health, U. S. Department of Health and Human Services. "Heart Disease and Hispanic Americans." Retrieved August 22, 2013, from http://minorityhealth.hhs.gov/.

———. "HIV/AIDS and Hispanic Americans." Retrieved August 22, 2013, from http://minorityhealth.hhs.gov/.

Office of Women's Health, U. S. Department of Health and Human Services. "Minority Women's Health, Latinas, Breast Cancer." Retrieved August 22, 2013, from http://womenshealth.gov/.

Ogden, C. L., M. D. Carroll, B. K. Kit, and K. M. Flegal. "Prevalence of Obesity and Trends in Body Mass Index among US Children and Adolescents, 1999–2010." *Journal of the American Medical Association* 307, no. 5 (2012): 483–90.

Orfield, G., and J. T. Yun. "Resegregation in American Schools." The Civil Rights Project, Harvard University. Available at: www.law.harvard.edu/.

Ortiz de Montellano, B. R. *Aztec Medicine, Health, and Nutrition.* New Brunswick, NJ: Rutgers University Press, 1990.

Padilla, A. M., and V. N. Salgado de Snyder. "Hispanics: What the Culturally Informed Evaluator Needs to Know." In *Cultural Competence for Evaluators: A Guide for Alcohol and Other Drug Abuse Prevention Practitioners Working with Ethnic/Racial Communities*, ed. M. A. Orlandi, R. Weston, and L. G. Epstein, 117–46. Rockville, MD: U.S. Department of Health and Human Services, Public Health Service, Alcohol, Drug Abuse, and Mental Health Administration, 1992.

Padilla, E. R., and A. M. Padilla, eds. *Transcultural Psychiatry: An Hispanic Perspective.* Spanish Speaking Mental Health Research Center Monograph No. 4. Los Angeles: University of California at Los Angeles, 1977.

Palerm, Juan Vicente, and Matt T. Salo. "Immigrant and Migrant Farm Workers in the Santa Maria Valley, California,." U.S. Census Bureau Research Report #EX95/21, 1995. Available at: http://www.census.gov/.

Park, J., and J. S. Buechner. "Race, Ethnicity, and Access to Health Care, Rhode Island." *Journal of Health and Social Policy* 9, no. 1 (1997): 1–14.

Portes, A., and A. Stepick. "A Repeat Performance? The Nicaraguan Exodus." In *Challenging Fronteras: Structuring Latina and Latino Lives in the United States*, ed. M. Romero, P. Hondagneu-Sotelo, and V. Ortiz, 135–51. New York: Routledge, 1997.

Public Broadcasting Service. *AZ House Bill 2281.* Retrieved on November 13, 2014, from http://www.pbs.org/.

Pulido, L. *Environmentalism and Economic Justice: Two Chicano Struggles in the Southwest.* Tucson: University of Arizona Press, 1996.

Raffaelli, M., and L. L. Ontai. "Gender Socialization in Latino/a Families: Results from Two Retrospective Studies." *Sex Roles* 50 (2004): 287–99.

Rapoport, J., R. L. Robertson, and B. Stuart. *Understanding Health Economics.* Rockville, MD: Aspen Publications, 1982.

Reference for Business. "Medicare and Medicaid." In *Encyclopedia of Business*, 2nd ed. Retrieved on November 19, 2010, from http://www.referenceforbusiness .com/.

Reichman, J. S. "Language-Specific Response Patterns and Subjective Assessment of Health: A Sociolinguistic Analysis." *Hispanic Journal of Behavioral Sciences* 19, no. 3 (August 1997): 353–68.

Rodríguez, S. "The Hispano Homeland Debate Revisited." *Perspectives in Mexican American Studies* 3 (1992): 95–114.

Rodríguez-Trias, H., and A. B. Ramírez de Arellano. "The Health of Children and Youth." Chapter 5 in *Latino Health in the United States: A Growing Challenge*, ed. C. W. Molina and M. Aguirre-Molina. Washington, DC: American Health Association, 1994.

Romero, M., P. Hodagneu-Sotelo, and V. Ortiz. *Challenging Fronteras*. New York and London: Routledge, 1997.

Schu, C. L., M. L. Burc, C. D. Good, and E. N. Gardner. *California's Undocumented Latino Immigrants: A Report on Access to Health Care Services*. Bethesda, MD: The Project HOPE Center for Health Affairs, 1999.

Segura, D. A., and A. de la Torre. "La Sufrida: Contradictions of Acculturation and Gender in Latina Health." In *Revisioning Women, Health, and Healing*, ed. A. E. Clarke and V. L. Oleson. New York and London: Routledge, 1999.

Selik, R. M., K. G. Castro, and M. Pappaioanou. "Racial/Ethnic Differences in the Risk of AIDS in the United States." *American Journal of Public Health* 78 (1988): 1539–45.

Shaefer, H. L., C. M. Grogan, and H. A. Pollack. "Transitions from Private to Public Health Coverage among Children: Estimating Effects on Out-Of-Pocket Medical Costs and Health Insurance Premium Costs." *Health Services Research* 46, no. 3 (2011): 840–58.

Shaefer, H. L., and E. D. Sammons. "The Development of an Unequal Social Safety Net: A Case Study of Employer-Based Health Insurance (Non) System." *Journal of Sociology and Social Welfare* 36, no. 3 (2009): 179–99.

Singer, M. "Confronting the AIDS Epidemic among IV Drug Users: Does Ethnic Culture Matter?" *AIDS Education and Prevention* 3, no. 3 (1991): 258–83.

———. "A Dose of Drugs, a Touch of Violence, a Case of AIDS: Conceptualizing the SAVA Syndemic." *Free Inquiry in Creative Sociology* 24, no. 2 (1996): 99–110.

Social Security Administration website: http://www.ssa.gov/; search keyword SSI.

Sparks, S. N., R. Tisch, and M. Gardner. "Family-Centered Interventions for Substance Abuse in Hispanic Communities," *Journal of Ethnicity in Substance Abuse* 12 (2013): 68–81.

State of Arizona House of Representatives, Forty-ninth Legislature (2010). HB 2281. S. o. A. H. o. Representatives. http://www.azleg.gov/.

State of California, Department of Health Care Services, *Medi-Cal Program Enrollment Totals for Fiscal Year 2008–09*. Retrieved on November 22, 2010, from http://www.dhcs.ca.gov/.

Stevens, S. J., J. R. Erickson, and A. L. Estrada. "Characteristics of Female Sexual Partners of Injection Drug Users in Southern Arizona: Implications for Effective HIV Risk Reduction Interventions." *Drugs and Society* 7, no. 3/4 (1993): 129–42.

Substance Abuse and Mental Health Services Administration. *Data from the Drug Abuse Warning Network* (DAWN). 1994 Data File. Rockville, MD: SAMHSA, 1994.

———. *Results from the 2009 National Survey on Drug Use and Health: Volume I. Summary of National Findings*. Office of Applied Studies, NSDUH Series H-38A, HHS Publication No. SMA 10–4586 Findings. Rockville, MD, 2010.

Substance Abuse and Mental Health Services Administration, Office of Applied Studies. *Drug Abuse Warning Network, 2007: National Estimates of Drug-Related Emergency Department Visits*. Rockville, MD, 2010. https://dawninfo.samhsa.gov/.

———. October 29, 2009. *The NSDUH Report: Injection Drug Use and Related Risk Behaviors*. Rockville, MD. Retrieved on November 13, 2010, from http://oas.samhsa.gov/.

———. 1998. *Prevalence of Substance Use among Racial and Ethnic Subgroups in the U.S.* Retrieved on November 13, 2010, from http://oas.samhsa.gov/.

Sundquist, J., and M. A. Winkleby. "Cardiovascular Risk Factors in Mexican American Adults: A Transcultural Analysis of NHANES III, 1988–1994." *American Journal of Public Health* 89, no. 5 (1999): 723–30.

Texas A&M University website: http://resi.tamu.edu/.

Texas Department of Human Services website: www.dhs.state.tx.us/programs/TexasWorks/pregnant.html.

Timmreck, T. C. *Health Services Cyclopedic Dictionary*, 3rd ed. Boston: Jones and Bartlett Publishers, 1997.

Triandas, H. C. *The Analysis of Subjective Culture*. New York: John Wiley, 1972.

University of Indiana drug prevention resource website: http://www.drugs.indiana.edu/.

UPI. "Study: Risk of Coronary Disease Higher in Hispanics." UPI Science Report, November 8, 1998.

U.S. Census Bureau website: http://www.census.gov/.

U.S. Census Bureau. *Current Population Survey, March 1997*. Washington, DC: Government Printing Office, 1997.

———. *Current Population Survey, Annual Social and Economic (ASEC)*. Supplement, 2009. Washington, DC: Government Printing Office, 2010. Retrieved on November 19, 2010, from http://www.census.gov/.

———. "Hispanic Americans By the Numbers." Retrieved August 22, 2013, from http://www.infoplease.com/.

———. "2010 Census Interactive Population Search: Texas." Retrieved August 22, 2013, from http://www.census.gov/.

———. "2010 Census Interactive Population Search: New Mexico." Retrieved August 22, 2013, from http://www.census.gov/.

U.S. Census Bureau, Current Population Reports, P60-238, *Income, Poverty, and Health Insurance Coverage in the United States: 2009*, by C. DeNavas-Walt, B. D. Proctor, and J. C. Smith. Washington, DC: Government Printing Office, 2010.

———. *Census of Population.* Washington, DC: Government Printing Office, 1990.

———. *Health Insurance Coverage: 1997*, Current Population Reports, Series P60–202. Washington, DC: Government Printing Office, September 1998.

U.S. Citizenship and Immigration Services (2012, August 15, 2013). "E-Verify." Retrieved August 22, 2013, from http://www.uscis.gov/.

U.S. Department of Health and Human Services, Public Health Service and Health Resources and Services Administration, *Health Status of Minorities and Low-Income Groups*, 3rd ed. Washington, DC: Government Printing Office, 1991.

U.S. Department of Justice, Drug Enforcement Administration website: www.usdoj.gov/dea/.

Vargas, R., and S. Martínez. *Razalogía: Community Learning for a New Society.* Oakland, CA: Razagente Associates, 1984.

Velasco, A. *Finding, Interviewing, and Retrieving Blood Samples from Tecatos: AIDS Prevention and Research in San Diego.* DHHS Pub. No. (ADM) 91–1752, pp. 121–25. Washington, DC: U.S. Department of Health and Human Services, 1991.

Webster's Third New International Dictionary of the English Language, Unabridged. Springfield, MA: Merriam-Webster, 1986.

Williams, S. J., and P. R. Torrens. *Introduction for Health Services.* 2nd ed. New York: Wiley, 1984.

Yahoo Insurance Glossary website: http://gen.insweb.yahoo.com/.

Youth Risk Behavior Survey. Atlanta, GA: CDC, 1995.

Yu, H., and A. W. Dick. "Impacts of Rising Health Care Costs on Families with Employment-based Private Insurance: A National Analysis with State Fixed Effects." *Health Services Research* 47 (5): 2012–30.

Zambrana, M. M. *Mejor Sola que Mal Acompañada: For the Latina in an Abusive Relationship.* Seattle: The Seal Press, 1985.

INDEX

Page numbers followed by *f* refer to figures; page numbers followed by *t* refer to tables.

proteinuria, 59
psychological inoculation, 92

Quiñones, Lily, 8, 17
Quiroga, Marissia, 17, 105

racialized labor markets, 7
racial profiling, 11. *See also* discrimination; racism
racism, 30, 35–40, 138–39, 143–44, 156. *See also* discrimination; racial profiling
razalogía model, 50–51
relative risk, 48–49
religiosity, 50
respeto, 10, 47, 50, 154
reverse language shifts, 29–31
Rochín, Refugio, 17, 19

Saenz, Graciela Guzmán, 6, 18, 19, 33, 64–65, 132–33, 141–42
salmon bias hypothesis, 68–69
Salud Migrante, 120
SCHIP (State Children's Health Insurance Program), 107
school dropouts. *See* dropouts
segregation, 34–35, 40
seniors, 114–15
sexuality, 56, 63, 86–87
sexually transmitted diseases (STDs), 56, 63. *See also* HIV/AIDS
simpatía, 50
smoking. *See* tobacco use
sobadoras, 135
social location, 3–4
socioeconomic status, 6–9, 46–47, 50–52, 55, 68. *See also* educational attainment; income; occupational location
Spanish explorers, 45, 69

spirituality, 50
spousal abuse. *See* intimate partner violence
SSI (Supplemental Security Income), 106–7
State Children's Health Insurance Program (SCHIP), 107
STDs (sexually transmitted diseases), 56, 63. *See also* HIV/AIDS
strokes, 59
subjective culture, 50
substance abuse: acculturation and nativity factors, 82–83; deaths and, 89–90; emergency room visits, 88–89; HIV/AIDS and, 84–88, 93–94; individual and interpersonal factors, 80–82; injection drug use, 10, 76, 78, 84–86; Latinos/Latinas and, 76–79; morbidity and mortality, 90; overview, 8–10; prevention, 90–92; social context and, 79–80; violent crimes and, 83–84
suicides, 56
Supplemental Security Income (SSI), 106–7

teen pregnancy, 56, 154
Teyolia, 44–45
therapeutic treatment models, 143–44, 156
tobacco use, 64, 81, 90
Tonalli, 44–45
tooth decay. *See* oral health
Treaty of Guadalupe Hidalgo, 24, 27
Type II diabetes. *See* non-insulin-dependent diabetes

UC PRIME program, 12, 124, 155
undocumented immigrants, 118–21, 155

ABOUT THE AUTHORS

Adela de la Torre, an agricultural and health economist, is vice chancellor of Student Affairs, professor of Chicana/o Studies, and director of the Center for Transnational Health at the University of California, Davis. She received her PhD in agricultural and resource economics from the University of California, Berkeley, and completed her health policy postdoctoral training at the Institute for Health Policy Studies at the University of California, San Francisco. Her publications and research focus on health care and educational disparities that affect the Latino/a community. Her most recent research project is Niños Sanos, Familia Sana, a multi-intervention study to prevent childhood obesity in Mexican-origin children in rural California funded by USDA-NIFA. Her NIH- and NSF-funded research includes developing institutional and local strategies to improve the educational success of Latinos and increase diversity in K–12 and higher education.

Antonio Estrada is professor of Mexican American Studies, medicine, and public health at the University of Arizona. Estrada received his PhD and MS degrees in public health with training in behavioral sciences/health education, social epidemiology, and evaluation research from the UCLA School of Public Health. Estrada's research interests include HIV disease among injection-drug users and their sexual partners, prevention with HIV positives, and Hispanic/Latino health disparities. He has been the principal investigator on two R01 research grants and an NIH minority supplement, has served as co-principal investigator on three NIH-funded grants, and has received state and private foundation funding for his research. Estrada has also been employed as the chief evaluator for two multisite HRSA Special Projects of National Significance (SPNS) focused on prevention with HIV-positive persons and increasing access to medical care among HIV positive persons in the U.S.-Mexico border region.